# BITS & BYTES

## *Surviving Morning Rounds*

A.B.R. Thomson

*Disclaimer: Neither the author(s) nor CAPStone Academic Publishers can ensure the accuracy of the information contained in these books with regards to regional variations for recommended indications, dosages, and reportable adverse events. With the rapid expansion of medical knowledge, there may be, from time to time, variations between what is published in these books and the latest information and consensus recommendations made by different organizations. It is the responsibility of the reader to confirm independently any practice decisions related to an individual patient.*

# BITS & BYTES

## *Surviving Morning Rounds*

**A.B.R. Thomson**

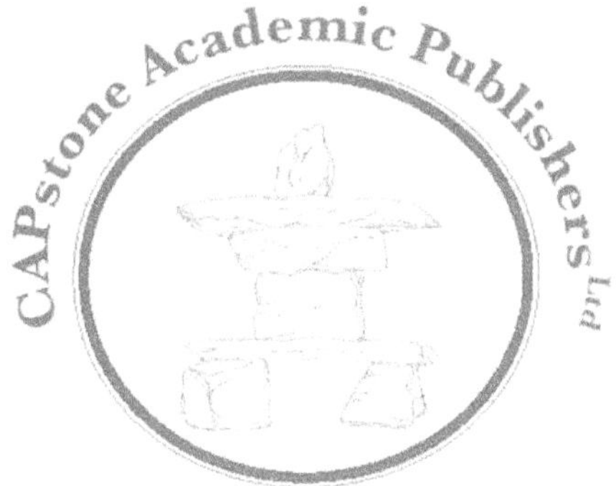


*CAPstone (Canadian Academic Publishers Ltd) is a not-for-profit company dedicated to the use of the power of education for the betterment of all persons everywhere.*

*"The Democratization of Knowledge"*
*2012*

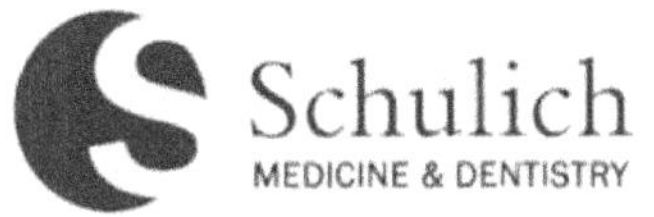


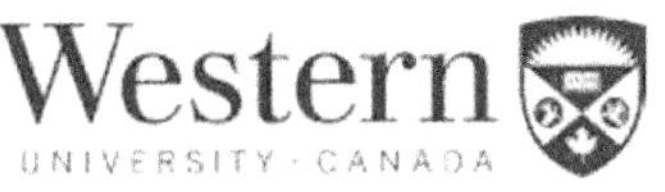


# THE WESTERN WAY

## Table of contents

"A man sooner or later discovers that
he is the master-gardener of his soul,
the director of his life"

James Allen

## Bits & Bytes and the CANMED Objectives

**Medical expert**
The discussion of complex cases provides the participants with an opportunity to comment on additional focused history and physical examination. They would provide a complete and organized assessment. Participants are encouraged to identify key features, and they develop an approach to problem-solving.

The case discussions, as well as the discussion of cases around a diagnostic imaging, pathological or endoscopic base provides the means for the candidate to establish an appropriate management plan based on the best available evidence to clinical practice. Throughout, an attempt is made to develop strategies for diagnosis and development of clinical reasoning skills.

**Communicator**
The participants demonstrate their ability to communicate their knowledge, clinical findings, and management plan in a respectful, concise and interactive manner. When the participants play the role of examiners, they demonstrate their ability to listen actively and effectively, to ask questions in an open-ended manner, and to provide constructive, helpful feedback in a professional and non-intimidating manner.

**Collaborator**
The participants use the "you have a green consult card" technique of answering questions as fast as they are able, and then to interact with another health professional participant to move forward the discussion and problem solving. This helps the participants to build upon what they have already learned about the importance of collegial interaction.

**Manager**
The participants are provided with assignments in advance of the three day GI Practice Review. There is much work for

them to complete before as well as afterwards, so they learn to manage their time effectively, and to complete the assigned tasks proficiently and on time. They learn to work in teams to achieve answers from small group participation, and then to share this with other small group participants through effective delegation of work. Some of the material they must access demands that they use information technology effectively to access information that will help to facilitate the delineation of adequately broad differential diagnoses, as well as rational and cost effective management plans.

**Health advocate**

In the answering of the questions and case discussions, the participants are required to consider the risks, benefits, and costs and impacts of investigations and therapeutic alliances upon the patient and their loved ones.

**Scholar**

By committing to the pre- and post-study requirements, plus the intense three day active learning Practice Review with colleagues is a demonstration of commitment to personal education. Through the interactive nature of the discussions and the use of the "green consult card", they reinforce their previous learning of the importance of collaborating and helping one another to learn.

**Professional**

The participants are coached how to interact verbally in a professional setting, being straightforward, clear and helpful. They learn to be honest when they cannot answer questions, make a diagnosis, or advance a management plan. They learn how to deal with aggressive or demotivated colleagues, how to deal with knowledge deficits, how to speculate on a missing knowledge byte by using first principals and deductive reasoning. In a safe and supportive setting they learn to seek and accept advice, to acknowledge awareness of personal limitations, and to give and take 360° feedback.

**Knowledge**

The basic science aspects of gastroenterology are considered in adequate detail to understand the mechanisms of disease, and the basis of investigations and treatment. In this way, the participants respect the importance of an adequate foundation in basic sciences, the basics of the design of clinical research studies to provide an evidence-based approach, the designing of clinical research studies to provide an evidence-based approach, the relevance of their management plans being patient-focused, and the need to add “compassionate” to the Three C’s of Medical Practice: competent, caring and compassionate.

“They may forget what you said, but they will never forget how you made them feel.”

Carl W. Buechner, on teaching.

“With competence, care for the patient. With compassion, care about the person.”

Alan B. R. Thomson, on being a physician.

## Prologue

HREs, better known as, High Risk Examinations. After what is often two decades of study, sacrifice, long hours, dedication, ambition and drive, we who have chosen Internal Medicine, and possibly through this a subspecialty, have a HRE, the [Boards] Royal College Examinations. We have been evaluated almost daily by the sadly subjective preceptor based assessments, and now we face the fierce, competitive, winner-take-all objective testing through multiple choice questions (MCQs), and for some the equally challenging OSCE, the objective standardized clinical examination. Well we know that in the real life of providing competent, caring and compassionate care as physicians, as internists, that a patient is neither a MCQ or an OSCE. These examinations are to be passed, a process with which we may not necessarily agree. Yet this is the game in which we have thus far invested over half of our youthful lives. So let us know the rules, follow the rules, work with the rules, and succeed. So that we may move on to do what we have been trained to do, do what we may long to do, care for our patients.

The process by which we study for clinical examinations is so is different than for the MCQs: not trivia, but an approach to the big picture, with thoughtful and reasoned deduction towards a diagnosis. Not looking for the answer before us, but understanding the subtle aspects of the directed history and focused physical examination, yielding an informed series of hypotheses, a differential diagnosis to direct investigations of the highly sophisticated laboratory and imaging procedures now available to those who can wait, or pay.

This book provides clinically relevant questions of the process of taking a history and performing a physical examination, with sections on Useful background, and where available, evidence-based performance characteristics of the rendering of our clinical skills. Just for fun are included "So you want to be a such-and-such specialist!" to remind us that one if the greatest strengths we can possess to survive in these times, is to smile and even to laugh at ourselves.

Sincerely,

Alan Thomson

Emeritus Distinguished University Professor,
University of Alberta

Adjunct Professor, Western University

## Dedication

To my grandparents, Grace (Jordan) and Arthur Lewis,

And to my Baba and Papa, Nadja (Sak Rewskaja) and Nicholaj Stecenko

"I thought of you with love today"
Anonymous

**Acknowledgements**

Patience and patients go hand in hand. So also does the interlocking of young and old, love and justice, equality and fairness. No author can have thoughts transformed into words, no teacher can make ideas become behaviour and wisdom and art, without those special people who turn our minds to the practical - of getting the job done!

Thank you, Naiyana and Duen for translating those terrible scribbles, called my handwriting, into the still magical legibility of the electronic age. Thank you, Sarah, for your creativity and hard work.

My most sincere and heartfelt thanks go to the excellent persons at JP Consulting, and CapStone Academic Publishers. Jessica, you are brilliant, dedicated and caring. Thank you.

When Rebecca, Maxwell, Megan Grace, Henry and Felix ask about their Grandad, I will depend on James and Anne, Matthew and Allison, Jessica and Matt, and Benjamin to be understanding and kind. For what I was trying to say and to do was to make my professional life focused on the three C's - competence, caring, and compassion - and to make my very private personal life dedicated to family - to you all.

**ARE YOU PREPARING FOR EXAMS IN GASTROENTEROLOGY AND HEPATOLOGY?**

See the full range of examination preparation and review publications from CAPstone on Amazon.com

Gastroenterology and Hepatology

- First Principles of Gastroenterology and Hepatology, 6th edition (ISBN: 978-1461038467)
- GI Practice Review, 2nd edition (ISBN: 978-1475219951)
- Endoscopy and Diagnostic Imaging Part I (ISBN: 978-1477400579)
- Endoscopy and Diagnostic Imaging Part II (ISBN: 978-1477400654)
- Scientific Basis for Clinical Practice in Gastroenterology and Hepatology (ISBN: 978-1475226645)

General Internal Medicine

- Achieving Excellence in the OSCE. Part I. Cardiology to Nephrology (ISBN: 978-1475283037)
- Achieving Excellence in the OSCE. Part II. Neurology to Rheumatology (ISBN: 978-1475276978)
- Mastering the Boards and Clinical Examinations. Part I. Cardiology, Endocrinology, Gastroenterology, Hepatology and Nephrology (ISBN: 978-1461024842)
- Mastering the Boards and Clinical Examinations. Part II. Neurology to Rheumatology (ISBN: 978-1478392736)

## Cardiology

### 1. Aorta

Q1. What are the *types of aortic coarctation*?

A1. ➢ Common:

- Infantile or preductal where the aorta between the left subclavian artery and patent ductus arteriosus is narrowed. Its manifests in infancy with heart failure. Associated lesions include patent ductus arteriosus, aortic arch anomalies, transposition of the great arteries, ventricular septal defect.
- Adult type: the coarctation in the descending aorta is juxtaductal or slightly postductal. It may be associated with bicuspid aortic valve or patent ductus arteriosus. It commonly between the age of 15 and 30 years.

➢ Rare

- Localized juxtaductal corctation
- Coarctation of the ascending thoracic aorta

Source: Baliga RR. *Saunders/Elsevier* 2007, page 85.

Q2. Young persons may be diagnosed with coarctation of the aorta, whereas in older persons aortic disease may be from dissection or obstruction from atherosclerosis. What abnormalities found on *physical examination* will suggest these diseases of the aorta?

A2. ○ Asymmetry

- R. vs L. arm
- Arm vs Leg

} - Pulse strength, timing
- Systolic blood pressure

Q3. What are the *complications* of aortic coarctation?

A3. o Severe hypertension and resulting complications:

- Stroke
- Premature coronary artery disease

Q4. What are the *findings in the fundus* of the eye in coarctation of aorta?

A4. Hypertension due to coarctation of aorta causes retinal arteries to be tortuous with frequent 'U' turns; curiously, the classical signs of hypertensive retinopathy are rarely seen.

Source: Baliga RR. *Saunders/Elsevier* 2007, page 87.

## 2. Aortic stenosis (AS)

Q1. From the palpation of a central artery (brachial or carotid), *differentiate* between supravalvular aortic stenosis versus either subvalvular or valvular aortic stenosis?

A1.

| Supravalvular | Subvalvular |
| --- | --- |
| o Rapid upstroke | o Slow upstroke |
| o ↑ Pulse pressure | o ↓ pulse pressure |
| o ↓ duration of peak (summit) | o ↑ duration of peak |

Adapted from: Mangione S. *Hanley & Belfus* 2000, page 183.

Q2. In the presence of aortic stenosis (AS) or hypertrophic cardiomyopathy (HC), what is the *Brockenbrough-Braunwald- Morrow* (B-B-M) sign?

A2. A fall in pulse pressure after an extrasystolic beat.

Q3. What is the difference between the brachial *pulse* in ventricular versus supraventricular aortic stenosis (AS)?

A3. In ventricular AS, R=L brachial pulse. In supraventricular AS, the left brachial pulse has slow uptake (pulsus tardus), but the right brachial pulse is normal (L < R).
Source: Mangione S. *Hanley & Belfus* 2000, page 182.

Q4. In which types of *muscular dystrophy* is myocardial involvement most frequent?

A4.
- Pseudohypertrophic muscular dystrophy
- Dystrophia myotonia

Q5. How would you *differentiate* aortic stenosis (AS) from aortic sclerosis?

A5.
- Aortic sclerosis is seen in the elderly
- The pulse is normal volume
- The apex beat is not shifted
- The murmur is localized

Q6. How does the patient's age affect the likely *cause* of their aortic stenosis?

A6.
- Under the age of 60 years: rheumatic, congenital.
- Between 60 and 75 years: calcified bicuspid aortic valve, especially in men.
- Over the age of 75 years: degenerative calcification

Source: Baliga RR. *Saunders/Elsevier* 2007, page 19.

### 3. Aortic Regurgitation (AR)

Q1. The early diastolic murmur of AR is usually heard best with the diaphragm and at the LSE. What is the *significance* of this murmur being auscultated at both the right and the left sternal edge?

A1. As a result of the AR, the ascending aorta becomes dilated and displaced, so that this high pitched early diastolic murmur becomes audible on both sides of the sternum.

Q2. Stump Your Staff – See if they know more than four of the *eponymous signs* of aortic regurgitation

A2.

- Quincke's sign: capillary pulsation in the nail beds- it is of no value, as this sign occurs normally
- Corrigan's sign: prominent carotid pulsations
- De Musset's sign: head nodding in time with the heartbeat
- Hill sign: increased blood pressure in the legs compared with the arms
- Mueller's sign: pulsation of the uvula in time with the heartbeat
- Duroziez sign: systolic and diastolic murmurs over the femoral artery on gradual compression of the vessel
- Traube's sign: a double sound heard over the femoral artery on compressing the vessel distally; this is not a 'pistol shot' sound that may be heard over the femoral
- Corrigans neck pulsation
- De Mussetts head nodding
- Duroziez's femoral diastolic murmur
- Quincke's capillary pulsation (nails)

Source: Talley NJ, et al. *Maclennan & Petty Pty Limited* 2003, Table 3-13, page 78.

Q3. Under what circumstances is the blood pressure *lower in the legs* than arms (normal difference: 10-15 mm Hg higher in legs than arms)?

A3.
- Abnormal difference (Hill sign, > 20 mm Hg; exaggeration of normal, indicating ↑ SV (stroke volume)' such as from tachycardia
- Atherosclerosis in the elderly
- Aortic dissection
- Aortic regurgitation (severe)

Adapted from: Baliga RR. *Saunders/Elsevier* 2007, page 15.

Q4. In the setting of severe aortic regurgitation, what is *Duroziez' murmur*?

A4. Auscullation of the femoral artery with slowly increasing pressure of the diaphragm of the stethoscope on the artery causes a systolic and diastolic back – and – forth murmur.

Q5. The sensitivity of Duroziez maneuver for aortic regurgitation (AR) is 58 to 100%. Give 4 causes of *false negative Duroziez maneuver.*

A5.
- Mild AR
- AR plus AS
- AS plus MS (↓ LV filling from mitral stenosis [MS])
- AS plus MR (↓ LV emptying from mitral regurgitation [MR])
- Coarctation of the aorta

Q6. Perform a focused physical examination to distinguish between the Duroziez' double murmur of AR, and "*false positive*" *Duroziez sign*, not due to AR.

A6.
- This sign in AR is due to one murmur from forward flow, and one from reverse flow
- Any high – output state may cause a pulsus bisferiens as well as the Duroziez double murmur.
- The double murmur in high- outflow states, both due to forward flow
  - Auscultate over the femoral artery, and hear the to – and –fro murmur
  - Pressure over the cephalad edge of the compression stethoscope diaphragm increases both murmurs in high- output states
  - Pressure over the caudad edge of the diaphragm increases only the murmur from the reverse flow, as occurs in AR
- Distinction method

Cephalad pressure

↑ forward flow of both murmurs in high-output states

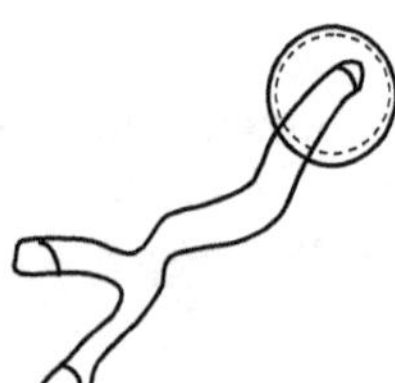

Caudad pressure

↑ reverse flow murmur position of the double murmur of AR

Q7. What causes *a systolic murmur* to accompany to the typical diastolic murmur of AR?

A7. Severe AR, or concurrent AS (i.e. AR+AS)

Q8. Aortic regurgitation (AR) has both a forward flow and a reverse flow component leading to the pulsus bisferiens and the "pistol shot" femoral bruit as well as the Duroziez' double murmur over the femoral artery. You auscultate a double murmur over the femoral artery, and pressure over the caudad portion of the *compressing* diaphragm of the stethoscope *enhances the reverse flow* murmur. But the patient does not have AR. What condition do they have?

A8. PDA (patent ductus arteriosus)

Q9. When a patient with AR was admitted, you discovered that she he had pulsus bisferiens. A week later the consultant cannot palpate this abnormal pulse. Did you *overcall* the presence of this abnormal pulse, because you knew they had AR and you thought they "should" have this kind of pulse?

A9. Not necessarily. The pulsus bisferiens lessens and then disappears when L-CHF develops.

Q10. In which cardiac phases are the *diagnosis and severity* of AR and MR made?

A10. Curious comparison: AR is diagnosed in diastole, but its severity assessed in systole; MR is diagnosed in systole, but its severity is assessed in diastole.

Q11. In the context of aortic regurgitation (AR), what is *Landolfi's sign*?

A11. The pupil contracts in systole, and dilates in diastole

Q12. In the context of aortic regurgitation, what is *"Hill sign*?"

A12.
- Higher systolic pressure in the leg than in the arm
- An indicator of the severity of aortic regurgitation

## 4. Arrhythmia

Q1. In the context of the patient with an arrhythmia, what is the "*holiday heart syndrome*" (HHS)?

A1.
- o Accentuation of the patients' disease when their cardiologist is away on vacation!
- o No!! HHS may occur when the chronic alcoholic goes as a binge of alcohol intake and develops a supraventricular arrhythmia.
- o There is a transient supraventicular arrhythmias (usually atrial fibrillation or atrial flutter) following an acute alcoholic binge in chronic alcoholics.

## 5. Atheroma, coronary arteries

Q1. The usual cause of ischemic heart disease (IHD) is atheroma in a coronary arteries. Give seven *other causes* of IHD, without or with narrowing.

A1.

| Without narrowing | With narrowing |
|---|---|
| o Inadequate blood supply<br>o Left ventricular hypertrophy<br>o ↓ blood supply to myocardium<br>- Aortic stenosis<br>- Mitral stenosis (severe)<br>- Pulmonary hypertension (severe) | o Embolism to coronary artery<br>- Atrial thrombi<br>- Air, fat emboli<br>- Embolization of vegetation from infected valve in SBE<br>o Congenital coronary artery fistula<br>o Polyarteritis nodosa, giant cell arteritis<br>o Syphilis (ostial stenosis, i.e. narrowing or origins of coronary artery) |

## 6. Congenital heart disease

Q1. What do Turner syndrome, Noonan syndrome and Bonnevie-Ullrich syndrome have in common?

A1. Webbed neck. Now let's consider further these three conditions.

- Turner syndrome
    - Phenotypic females
    - Cvarian dysgenesis
    - Short stature
    - Low-set ears
    - "shield chest|
    - Café-au-lait spots
    - Freckles
    - Heart congenital coarctation of aorta
- Bonnevie- Ullrich syndrome
    - Lymphedena of hands & feet
    - Nail dystrophy
    - Lax skin
    - Short stature
- Noonan syndrome
    - Congenital pulmonary stenosis
    - Pectus carinatum (forward projection of sternum
    - Short stature
    - Mildly mentally challenged
    - Hypertelevision
    - Bleeding
    - Skin changes

Q2. What are the *commonest types* of congenital heart disease?

A2.
- VSD (ventricular septal defect)
- ASD (atrial septal defect, secundum type)
- Fallot tetralogy

Q3. Under what clinical circumstances should heart disease be suspected as being *congenital* in origin?

A3.
- o Young person
- o Murmur down left sterna edge
- o Presence of both cyanosis and clubbing
- o Presence of other congenital conditions:
  - Down syndrome : ASD (ostium primuim type of atrial septal defect)
  - Turner syndrome: coarctation of the aorta, pulmonary stenosis
  - Gargoylism: fibroelastosis
  - Marfan syndrome : ASA, dissecting aneurysm

- o Depending upon underlying history, presence of
  - Cyanosis
  - Clubbing
  - Polycythemia (secondary to low pO2)
  - Drawfism, or infantilism (retention in adult life of sexual characteristics of childhood)

Q4. Congenital heart disease may be cyanotic or non-cyanotic in nature. What is *cyanosis tardive*?

A4. Persons with a congenital shunt (PDA, VSD, ASD) have the potential to develop cyanosis when the shunt reverses secondary to

- o CHF
- o Pulmonary infection
- o Exercise

Q5. What are the congenital disorders in which *atrial fibrillation* is common

A5.
- o Atrial septal defect (ASD)
- o Ebstein anomaly

Source: Baliga RR. *Saunders/Elsevier* 2007, pages 32 and 33.

Q6. In the context of ASD, what is the "*Lutembacher complex*"? What is the significance of this physical finding to the prognosis of the associated murmur?

A6. The lutembacher complex is ASD plus mitral stenosis (MS). When MS occurs with ASD, its prognosis is better than MS by itself.

Q7. What are the types of VSD?

A7.

- The supracristal type (above the crista supraventricularis):
  - A high defect just below the pulmonary valve and the right coronary cusp of the aortic valve
  - The latter may not be adequately supported, resulting in aortic regurgitation
  - In Fallot tetralogy this defect is associated with the rightward shift of the interventricular septum
  - In double-outlet left ventricle with subaortic stenosis the supracristal defects associated with a leftward shift of the septum

- The infracristal defect, which may be in either the upper membranous portion of the interventricular septum, or the lower muscular part
  - Small defects (maladie de Roger; curiously, a very loud murmur)
  - Swiss cheese appearance (multiple small defects)
  - Large defects
  - Gerbode defect (defect opening into the right atrium

Source: Baliga RR. *Saunders/Elsevier* 2007, page 169.

Q8. With regards a VSD, what is the "*Maladie de Roger*"?

A8. Maladie de Roger is a VSD with no hemodynamic consequences (no symptoms, no changes on chest X-ray or ECG).

Q9. With regards to a VSD, what is the importance of also auscultating a *mitral diastolic murmur* and a *pulmonary systolic murmur*?

A9. These murmurs are caused by an increase in the flow of blood through these mitral and pulmonary valves, indicating that the shunt is large and hemodynamically significant.

Q10. With regards to a VSD accompanied by a mitral diastolic murmur and a pulmonary systolic murmur, what is the hemodynamic significance of the *lessening* of these murmurs (loss of mitral murmur and lessening of pulmonary murmur)?

A10. With the increased blood flow through the mitral and pulmonary valves as the result of a large VSD shunt, the pressure in the right ventricle (RV) will increase and will reduce the flow which caused the murmurs.

Q11. In the context of a congenital or acquired VSD, what are *Graham Steell's murmur*, and Eisenmenger *complex*?

A11.

- Graham Steell's murmur - Murmur of PR (pulmonary regurgitation) in person with a VSD in which the flow through the defect decreases from the development of PHT, and the usual left - to- right shunting falls)
- Eisenmenger complex - The left - to – right flow in the VSD reverses with the development of pulmonary hypertension

Q12. What is the effect of *pregnancy* in women with VSD?

A12. Small defects should be present no problems.

Q13. Why does the hemodynamic *severity* of a VSD not reflect its size?

A13. The hemodynamic severity is reflected by the L → R shunt. The magnitude of this shunt may be reduced by

- ↑ pulmonary arteriolar resistance
- Hypertrophy of pulmonary outflow tract, leading to pulmonary stenosis (from functional muscular hypertrophic subvalvular pulmonary stenosis)

Q14. When does the typical pansystolic murmur of VSD occur *only in early systole*?

A14. The VSD is usually in the membranous portion of the ventricular septum. If the muscular part of the septum contracts, the murmur occurs only in early systole.

Q15. In the context of a continuous cardiac murmur present from birth, what lesion causes cyanosis and *clubbing of the toes, but not the hands*?

A15. Cyanosis and clubbing of the toes but not the hands is due to PDA.

Q16. Which congenital cardiac lesions are dependent on a *PDA*?

A16.
- Hypoplastic left heart syndrome
- Complex coarctations of aorta
- Critical congenital aortic stenosis

Q17. What happens to the *continuous murmur* of patent ductus arteriosus (PDA) in pulmonary hypertension?

A17. First the diastolic murmur, then the systolic murmur becomes softer and shorter and P2 increases in intensity

Source: Baliga RR. *Saunders/Elsevier* 2007, pages 78 and 81.

Q18. What happens to the continuous murmur of patent ductus arteriosus (PDA) in *pulmonary hypertension*?

A18.
- First the diatolic murmur, then the systolic murmur, becomes softer and shorter
- $P_2$ increases intensity

Source: Baliga RR. *Saunders/Elsevier* 2007, page 81.

Q19. Under what circumstances does the person with PDA develop cyanosis (*cyanosis tardive*)?

A19. With
- Exercise
- CHF
- Infection

Q20. Under what circumstances does the person with PDA develop *clubbing*?

A20. With
- SBE (subacute bacterial endocarditis)
- Pulmonary infection

Q21. What are the typical changes on the *chest X-ray* of the person with PDA?

A21.
- Large right atrium
- Large pulmonary conus and arteries ("hilar dance")
- Aorta normal size

Q22. What are the four *commonest causes* of cyanotic heart diseases of infancy?

A22. The Four T's:
- **T**etralogy of Fallot
- **T**ransposition of the great vessels
- **T**ricuspid regurgitation
- **T**otal anomalous pulmonary venous connection

Source: Baliga RR. *Saunders/Elsevier* 2007, page 89.

Q23. Give an example of a cyanotic cardiac condition where the *cyanosis* is more pronounced in the *feet* than in the hands.

A23. Eisenmenger's syndrome

Q24. Do you know all about Fallot and his *tetralogy*?

A24. Well, yes: ASD, pulmonary stenosis and right ventricular hypertrophy

Q25. Well then, what is Fallot's *pentatoly*?

A25. Fallot's tetralogy with associated ASD is known as Fallot's pentology

Source: Baliga RR. *Saunders/Elsevier* 2007, page 92.

Q26. What are the pathognomic "*Coeur de sabot*" findings on chest X-ray which suggest tetralogy of Fallot?

A26. Pathognomic

- o Aortic knuckle - normal
- o Pulmonary conus – concavity
- o Lower left heart border – upturned (due to RVH)
- o Hilum – enlarged right atrium and pulmonary artery
- o Lung fields – poorly seen

Abbreviation: RVH, right ventricular hypertrophy

Q27. What do you understand by the term '*situs inversus*'?

A27. Right-sided cardiac apex, right stomach, right-sided descending aorta. The right atrium is on the left. The left lung has three lobes and the right lung has two.

Q28. What do you understand by the term '*dextroversion*'?

A28. Right-sided cardiac apex, left sided stomach and left-sided descending aorta.

Q29. What do you understand by the term "*levoversion*'?

A29. Left-sided apex, right-sided stomach and right descending aorta

Source: Baliga RR. *Saunders/Elsevier* 2007, page 84.

Q30. What is *Kartagener's syndrome*?

A30. A type of immotile cilia syndrome in which there is dextrocardia situs inversus, bronchiectasis and dysplasia of the frontal sinuses.

Q31. Which *other abnormality* has been associated with dextrocardia?

A31. Asplenia (blood smear may show Heinz bodies, Howell-Jolly)

## 7. Congestive heart failure

Q1. In the context of wanting to pass the cardiology fellowship examination, what is "cor bovinum?"

A1. Slow and progressive left ventricular dilatation and hypertrophy in an attempt to normalize wall stress. The heart may thus become larger and heavier than in any other form of chronic heart disease – cor bovinum (bovine or ox heart)

Source: Baliga RR. *Saunders/Elsevier* 2007,page 15.

## 8. Coronary heart disease

Q1. In the context of coronary heart disease, what is *Dressler syndrom*e?

A1. Persistent pyrexia, pericarditis and pleurisy, post-myocardial infarction

Source: Baliga RR. *Saunders/Elsevier* 2007, pages 100 and 101.

Q2. What is the *cause and complication* of Dressler syndrome?

A2.
- Chest pain, pericardial effusion and fever occurring 3 weeks to 6 months after MI
- Complications include CHF and arrhythmias

## 9. Friedrich ataxia

Q1. What is Friedrich ataxia, and what are its associated *cardiac abnormalities*?

A1.
- Definition of Friedrich ataxia (FA)
  - CNS degeneration
    - Spinocerebellar tracts
    - Posterior columns
    - Pyramidal tracts
  - MSK abnormalities
    - Kyphoscoliosis
    - Pes cavis

- Cardiac abnormalities in FA
  - Cardiomegaly
  - Arrhythmias
  - Conduction defects

## 10. Heart sounds

- S2

Q1. If there is splitting of S2 during expiration, why do you *sit the patient up* and listen again?

A1. Splitting of S2 in expiration which disappears on sitting is normal, where as if splitting of S2 in expiration persists on sitting, then the wide, fixed or paradoxical splitting of S2 is abnormal.

Q2. What are the causes of *fixed splitting of S2* (splitting in both supine and sitting position?

A2.
- Severe CHF
- ASD
- VSD plus PHT (pulmonary hypertension)
- PS (pulmonary stenosis), PHT
- Massive PE

Adapted from: Mangione S. *Hanley & Belfus* 2000, pages 214 and 215.

Q3. Give the pathophysiological explanation for the cause of a *widely split* $S_2$ in the following conditions:

A3.

| | |
|---|---|
| ➢ ASD, VSD, PR | ○ ↑ RV volume |
| ➢ PS | ○ ↑ RV pressure |
| ➢ RBBB | ○ ↓ RV conduction |
| ➢ MR, VSD | ○ Early LV emptying |

Adapted from: Baliga RR. *Saunders/Elsevier* 2007, pages 72 and 73.

➢ S3

Q1. An $S_3$ is auscultated in a patient with a systolic murmur. There are no signs of associated CHF. What *prognostic value* does the $S_3$ have in terms of ventricular systolic dysfunction or increased filling pressure?

A1. In AS, but not in MR, $S_3$ reflects ventricular systolic dysfunction or increased filling pressure.

Q2. What is *the mechanism* of the production of S3?

A2. Caused by rapid ventricular filling in early diastole

Source: Baliga RR. *Saunders/Elsevier* 2007, page 39.

Q3. What are the *implications* of S3 in patients with valvular heart disease?

A3.
- In patients with mitral regurgitation, they are common but do not necessarily reflect ventricular systolic dysfunction or increase filling pressure
- In patients with aortic stenosis, third heart sounds are uncommon but usually indicate the presence of systolic dysfunction and raised filling pressure

Q4. What are the *causes* of the third heart sound ($S_3$)?

A4.
- Physiological: in normal children and young adults
- Pathological
  - Heart failure
  - Left ventricular dilatation without failure: mitral regurgitation, ventricular septal defect, patent ductus arteriosus
  - Right ventricular $S_3$ in right ventricular failure, tricuspid regurgitation

Q5. Does the fourth heart sound denote *heart failure*, like the $S_3$ gallop does?

A5. No

Source: Baliga RR. *Saunders/Elsevier* 2007, page 39.

- S4

Q1. What is the *relationship* between the intensity of $S_4$ and the severity of CHF?

A1. Dah, $S_4$ is not associated with CHF. If an elderly person has S4 plus CHF, the S4 is a normal finding in old age.

Q2. What are the *causes* of the fourth heart sound ($S_4$)?

A2.
- Normal: in the elderly
- Pathological:
  - Acute myocardial infarction
  - Aortic stenosis (the presence of $S_4$ in individuals below the age of 40 indicates significant obstruction)
  - Hypertension
  - Hyper trophic cardiomyopathy
  - Pulmonary stenosis

Adapted from: McGee SR. *Saunders/Elsevier* 2007, pages 217-225 and 434 to 437.

Q3. How do you *differentiate* between the fourth heart sound ($S_4$), a split first heart sound ($S_1$), and an ejection click?

A3. $S_4$ is not heard when pressure is applied on the chest piece of the strethoscope, but pressure does not eliminate the ejection sound or the slitting of the first heart sound.

Q4. What is the expression used when both the third and fourth heart sounds $S_3$ and $S_4$ are heard *with tachycardia*?

A4.
- The summation gallop
- Sometimes be mistaken for a diastolic rumbling murmur

Q5. What is the *difference* between “a snap”, “a click”, “a knock” and “a rub”?

A5.
- “Snap” – diastole, abnormal opening of the leaflets.
- “Click” – systole, prolapse and backward ballooning of valve leaflet(s).
- “Knock” (pericardial) - Louder and higher-pitched form of S3 (caused by early ventricular filling), and sudden stretching of the LV against a thick, calcified pericardium, or also heard in constrictive pericarditis. Occur in chronic calcified or constrictive pericarditis
- “Rub” (pericardial) - High-pitched, scratchy systolic and diastolic sounds, best heard with firm pressure of diaphragm, heard best at lower (3/4 interspaces) sterna border during inspiration, due to acute pericarditis

Source: Mangione S. *Hanley & Belfus* 2000, pages 225 to 236.

Q7. What does the $S_2$ tell us in *AS*?

A7.
- Normal: Strong evidence against the presence of critical aortic stenosis.
- Soft $S_2$. Valvular stenosis (except in calcific stenosis of the elderly, where the margins of the leaflets usually maintain their mobility)
- Single: Second heart sound may be heard when there is fibrosis and fusion of the valve leaflets
- Reversed splitting of the second sound: Indicates mechanical or electrical prolongation of ventricular systole.

Source: Baliga RR. *Saunders/Elsevier* 2007, page 19.

Q8. When does a *soft* $S_2$ occur in AS due to causes other than valvular stenosis?

A8. When the aortic valve is stenotic and is also calcified, if the leaflets remain mobile, $S_2$ may be soft but the stenosis is not valvular.

## 11. Hypertrophic cardiomyopathy (HOCM)

Q1. What are the *complications* of HOCM?

A1.
- Sudden death
- Atrial fibrillation
- Infective endocarditis
- Systemic embolization

Q2. What is the most *characteristic* pathophysiological abnormality in HOCM?

A2. Diastolic dysfunction

Source: Baliga RR. *Saunders/Elsevier* 2007, page 76.

## 12. Systemic hypertension

Q1. In primary hyperaldosteronism, what are the effects of variations in the *intake of salt* (NaCl) on aldosterone and rennin?

A1.
- High salt intake – no effect on aldosterone
- Low salt intake – no effect on renin

Q2. *Differentiate* between Pseudohypertension and Pseudohypotension

A2.
- Pseudohypertension – Artery can be palpated when a blood pressure cuff is inflated to the point of obliterating the radial pulse, and the artery is

still palpated as a firm tube in the absence of a pulse (Osler's maneuver). Positive Osler's sign, indicating the presence of arterosclerosis, and both SBP and DBP be overestimated.

- Pseudohypotension – in conditions of high peripheral vascular resistance such as shock, Korotkoff sounds are difficult to use to measure accurately systolic or diastolic pressure.

Source: Mangione S. *Hanley & Belfus* 2000, pages 28 and 29.

### 13. Mediastinal crunch

Q1. In the context of listening to the heart sounds, what is *Hamman Sign*?

A1.
- Crunching sound heard in time with systolic and diastolic components of heartbeat
- This "mediastinal crunch" is due to air in the mediastinum
- Seen after cardiac surgery, with a pneumothorax or aspiration of a pericardial effusion

Source: Talley NJ, et al. *Maclennan & Petty Pty Limited* 2003, page 59.

### 14. Mitral regurgitation (MR)

Q1. *Distinguish* between the murmur of MR due to RHD, from LV dilation and reduced contractility.

A1. MR from RHD: pansystolic murmur
MR from LV dilation: mid, late or pansystolic

Q2. *Distinguish* between the murmur of MR and AS with calcification.

A2. If there is a premature beat, or if there is associated AF, listen after the pause, when there is ↑ loudness of murmur in AS, but not in MR.

Abbreviation: AF, atrial fibrillation; AS, aortic stenosis; ASD, atrial septal defect; AV, atrioventricular; BV, blood volume; FP, filling pressure; LV, left ventricle; MR, mitral regurgitation; OS, opening snap; RHD, rheumatic heart disease; TR, tricuspid regurgitation; VSD, ventricular septal defect

Q3. In the context of MR, why does the peripheral pulse have *rapid upstroke* of short duration?

A3. ↑ BV regurgitating into LA causes ↓ LV ejection time.

Q4. The murmur of MR is usually associated with the apex beat displaced down and out. What is the mechanism by which the murmur of MR may *radiate to the neck*?

A4.
- If a stream of blood regurgitates from the LV into the LA near the aortic root, the murmur may radiate into the neck.
- This get of blood regurgitating to the aortic root may be seen with a ruptured cord as tendinae, or with disease involvement of the posterior leaflet of the mitral valve leaflet.

Q5. From the examination of the heart, how do you access the *severity* of MR?

A5. An $S_3$ suggests ↑ MR severity
A diastolic rumble (in the absence of associated MS) indicates ↑ BV flow across the mitral valve during diastole.

Q6. In the context of an systolic ejection murmur, what is the '*Gallavardin phenomenon*'?

A6. The high-frequency components of the ejection systolic murmur may radiate to the apex, falsely suggesting mitral regurgitation.

Source: Baliga RR. *Saunders/Elsevier* 2007, pages 32 and 33.

Q7. In the patient with combined MR and MS, (usually due to RHD), what is the significance of the *presence of an $S_3$ or a large LA*?

A7. MR + MS + $S_3$ – indicates the MS is mild, and the dominant murmur is the MR. MR + MS + large LA – same thing: MS is not clinically significant, and the main problem is the MS.

Source: Baliga RR. *Saunders/Elsevier* 2007, page 12.

Q8. In the patient with MR, what is the meaning of a *diastolic rumble*?

A8.
- MR+ MS (combined mitral disease)
- ↑ BV flow across the mitral valve during diastole

Q9. In persons with *mitral regurgitation* (MR), what is the meaning of a diastolic rumble?

A9. Coexistent mitral stenosis (MS)

Q10. In the patient with a thick chest, well aerated lung tissue and a large RV, even severe MR may not have an audible murmur of MR. How do you make the *diagnosis* of MR, in the absence of a murmur?

A10.
- Large L-atrium and L-ventricle
- $S_2$ widely split

Q11. When does the *absence* of a mitral area murmur or a late systolic/ holosystolic murmur significantly reduce the likelihood of mitral regurgitation?

A11. In the setting of an acute myocardial infarction.

Source: Simel DL, et al. *JAMA* 2009, page 439.

Q12. OK. In persons with MR, a diastolic rumble and a large left atrium, what is the interpretation?

A12. No associated MS

Source: Baliga RR. *Saunders/Elsevier* 2007, page 13.

Q13. You auscultate a systolic murmur which is suggestive of MR (mitral regurgitation). From the auscultation, how would you *distinguish* a MR murmur caused by (rheumatic heart disease), versus MVP (mitral valve prolapse) or PMA (papillary muscle dysfunction)?

A13. When

- RHD: platform murmur
- MVP or PMA
  - Systolic murmur of MR begins in mid-systole, and extends to $A_2$
  - Soft murmur, heard best at apex
  - Crescends pattern towards $S_2$
  - "Cooing" sound
  - "Honking" sound (like Canada geese)
  - Myxomatous degeneration of posterior leaflet
  - MVP syndrome:
    - Atypical chest pain
    - Arrhythmias
    - Abnormal ECG
  - Mimics PMD from MI or HOCM

- Sharp systolic click (chordal snap) in either mid or late systole, followed by murmur is typical of MVP, and can be made buder by exercise.

Adapted from: Mangione S. *Hanley & Belfus* 2000, pages 261 and 263.

Q14. Give the *causes* of a precordial pansystolic murmur.

A14.
- MR
- TR
- VSD

**15. Mitral stenosis (MS)**

Q1. The commonest cause of MS is RHD (Rheumatic heart disease). Give 4 *rare causes* of MS.

A1.
- Congenital
- Rheumatoid arthritis
- SLE
- Malignant carcinoid
- Mitral valve calcification

Abbreviation: SLE, systemic lupus erythematosis; MS, mitral stenosis

Q2. A mid-diastolic murmur is auscultated, and MS is suspected. Give the *differential* of the causes of a murmur which simulates MS.

A2.
- LA myxoma
- Ball valve thrombus of LA
- ASD
- Cor triatriatum (a membrane across the LA which partially blocks the pulmonary venous flow)

Q3. In the context of a mid-diastolic murmur which must be differentiated from MS, what is *Lutembacher syndrome*, and *Ortner syndrome*?

A3.
- Lutembacher syndrome : ASD + MS
- Ortner syndrome: Large LA in MS causing paralysis of left vocal cord, leading to hoarsensess.

Q4. A *tapping apex* beat in MS is caused by .....?

A4. A pronounced $S_1$.

Q5. *A loud $S_1$* in MS is caused by ...?

A5. Sudden closing of the valve leaflets during ventricular contraction in systole.

Q6. An *opening snap* in MS is caused by ...?

A6. Opening of the stenosed but pliable mitral valve leaflets.

Q7. In the patient with known MS, what is the implication of the *loss of the opening snap* (OS)?

A7. The OS is caused by the opening of the stenosed valve when the leaflets are pliable. Once the leaflets become calcified, the OS disappears.

Q8. The high-pitched OS occurs shortly after $S_2$, and the shorter the interval between $S_2$ and OS, the higher the LA pressure. What is the clinical significance of a *short interval* between $S_2$ and OS?

A8. A short interval between S2 and OS signifies ↑ LA pressure, and greater severity of MS.

Q9. The rumbling, low-pitched, mid-diastolic murmur of MS may be associated with presystolic accentuation. What is the *cause* of the presystolic accentuation, first when the patient is in sinus arythm, and secondly in *atrial fibrillation* (AF)?

A9.

- Sinus rhythm: increased flow during atrial systole across the narrowed.
- AF: turbulent flow across the mitral valve at the start of ventricular systole

Q10. What is the clinical significance of the diastolic murmur of MS becoming *softer*?

A10. When the stenosis across the mitral valve becomes tighter, the murmur becomes less prominent, even to the point of disappearing.

Q11. Give 3 findings suggesting that the MS is *severe*.

A11.

- Short distance between $S_2$ and OS
- Long duration of MS murmur
- Murmur of MS becoming softer
- Signs of pulmonary hypertension (PHT)

Q12. Perform a focused *physical examination* for PHT.

A12.
- ↑ $P_2$
- RV lift (L parasternal heave)
- ↑ JVP
- Ascites
- Peripheral edema
- Signs of etiology eg MS, COPD

Q13. What is the effect of *pregnancy* on MS?

A13.
- Patients usually become symptomatic in $T_2$
- Blood volume increases

Q14. In the context of MS, what is *Ortner syndrome*?

A14. Hoarseness of voice cause by keft vocal cord paralysis associated with enlarged left atrium in mitral stenosis

Source: Baliga RR. *Saunders/Elsevier* 2007, pages 4 and 7.

Q15. What causes the *tapping apex beat* in MS?

A15. An accentuated S1

Q16. What does a *soft S1* mean in MS?

A16. Loss of mobility of the valve leaflets

**16. Opening snap**

Q1. What does the opening snap *indicate*?

A1.
- Caused by the opening of the stenosed mitral valve and indicates that the leaflets are pliable

- Usually accompanied by a loud $S_1$
- Absent when the valve is diffusely calcified (when only the tips of the leaflets are calcified, the opening snap persists)

Source: Baliga RR. *Saunders/Elsevier* 2007, pages 4 and 7.

Q2. Give two circumstances when an *opening snap* does not occur with mitral stenosis (MS)

A2.
- Combined MS and MR (mitral regurgitation)
- Calcified mitral stenosis

**17. Mitral valve prolapsed (MVP)**

Q1. What is *the mechanism* of the click in MVP?

A1. Clicks result from sudden tensing of the mitral valve apparatus as the leaflets prolapse into the left atrium during systole.

Q2. In the context of a systolic murmur, what is the significance if after a long diastole (such as following a premature beat), the intensity of the murmur becomes *louder* at the base but not at the apex?

A2. Then the systolic murmur is likely comprised of both a regurgitation murmur plus an ejection murmur.

Q3. What is the *exception* to this general rule?

A3. The exception is mitral valve prolapse (MVP), in which, the murmur becomes softer after a long diastole.

**18. Orthopnea**

Q1. When does the person with chronic left sided (L) congestive heart failure lose their *orthopnea* (preferance to breathing in an upright position)?

A1.Once the L-CHF causes R-CHF, the failure of the RV causes unloading of the LV, relieving the pulmonary congestion.

Q2. 95% of persons with orthopnea will have heart disease, but what *pulmonary disease* makes up the remaining 5%?

A2. Bilateral, apical bullous disease (COPD)

**19.Pericarditis/ effusion/ rubs/ tamponade**

Q1. Which *2 causes* of pericardial rub do not usually progress to a pericardial effusion?

A1. Pericardial rub caused by myocardial infarction, or uremia.

Q2. What are the ECG changes which suggest that a rub has progressed to an *effusion*?

A2.
- o Low voltage
- o ↑ ST
- o Changes occur in all limb leads

Q3. What is the easy way *to distinguish* between the ECG changes of a myocardial infarction (MI) versus pericardial effusion?

A3. Low voltage and ↑ ST changes do not occur in all limb voltages in mL.

Q4. Which cause of constrictive pericarditis does not usually cause *cardiomegaly*, murmurs or atrial fibrillation (AF).

A4. Tuberculous pericarditis

Q5. In the context of cardiac tamponade, what is the *Beck triad*?

A5.
- Low arterial blood pressure
- High venous pressure
- Absent apex in cardiac tamponade is known as Beck triad

Source: Baliga RR. *Saunders/Elsevier* 2007, page 100.

Q6. In the context of the patient with constrictive pericarditis, what is Broadbent sign?

A6. Intercostal indrawing during systole.

**20. Pulmonary stenosis (PS)**

Q1. What are the *types* of PS?

A1.
- Valvular
- Subvalvular: infundibular and subinfundibular
- Supravalvular

Source: Baliga RR. *Saunders/Elsevier* 2007, page 82.

Q2. What are the *causes* of pulmonary stenosis?

A2.
- Congenital (commonest cause)
- Carcinoid tumor of the small bowel

Q3. How can valvular pulmonary stenosis (PS) be *distinguished* from on a chest X-ray?

A3. Only valvular PS has post-stenotic dilation.

## 21. Pulse pressure

Q1. What is the influence of the pulse pressure (PP) on the interpretation of the *palpation* of a rapid arterial upstroke?

A1.

- ↑ PP, rapid upstroke
  - Normal collapse
    - Mitral regurgitation
    - VSD
    - HOCM
  - Rapid collapse – aortic regurgitation
  - Hyperkinetic heart syndromes (high – output states)
- PP, rapid upstroke
  - Emptying into a low pressure area[1]
    - VSD
    - MR
  - Emptying into a high pressure area[2] - HOCM

1) rapid emptying of LV
2) LVH, delayed LV obstruction

Adapted from: Mangione S. *Hanley & Belfus* 2000, page 184.

Q2. In the context of increased pulse pressure in one limb (due to AV fistula), what is the area of the *Branham sign*? (compressing the area of suspected AV fistula causes ↓ HR).

A2. Branham sign is bradycardia caused by inhibiting the ↑ RA pressure caused by the fistula, thereby inhibiting vagal and stimulating the sympathetic pathway [Bainbridge reflex]).

**22. Peripheral pulses**

Q1. Palpation of the peripheral arterial pulse is a time-honoured part of the physical examination. Under what circumstances should you palpate the peripheral arteries on *both sides* of the body, the peripheral arteries in the *upper and lower* portions of the body, and the *carotid or brachial* arteries?

A1.
- Right and left sides, considering possible asymmetry
  - Thrombosis
  - Atherosclerosis
  - Embolism
  - Dissection
  - External compression/ occlusion
- Upper and lower peripheral arteries
  - In hypertension patient who may have coarctation of the aorta, or supravalvular aortic stenosis
- Central arteries
  - When trying to characterize the form of the arterial wave

Q2. What cardiac murmur is typically associated with a slow upstroke (*pulsus tardus*)?

A2. Pulsus tardus is associated with aortic stenosis.

Q3. Give three *mechanisms* for the development of pulsus parvis.

A3.

- Definition: pulsus parvis is a pulse with a low upstroke amplitude.
- Mechanisms for development of pulsus parvis
  - ↓ LV outflow, e.g. aortic stenosis
  - ↓ LV contraction, e.g. cardiomyopathy
  - ↓ LV filling, e.g. mitral stenosis

Q4. What is the difference in the cause of pulsus parvus by itself (↓ amplitude of upstroke, but upstroke otherwise normal), versus *pulsus parvus plus pulsus tardus* (slow uptake portion of arterial pulse)?

A4.

- Pulsus parvus, normal upstroke
  - ↓ LV contraction
  - ↓ LV filling
- Pulsus parvus and pulsus tardus
  - Aortic stenosis

Q5. What is the mechanism causing a *hyperkinetic pulse* in addition to ↑ speed of contraction & ↑ SV?

A5. ↓ Arterial compliance (especially in the presence of ↑ SBP)

Abbreviation: SBP, systolic blood pressure; SV, stroke volume

Q6. What is the *difference* between pulsus parvus plus tardis, versus hyperkinetic pulse?

A6.
- Pulsus parvus plus pulsus tardis (low amplitude plus slow upstroke) usually means presence of aortic stenosis
- Hyperkinetic pulse (rapid upstroke, high amplitude): wide pulse pressure, aortic regurgitation. Normal pulse pressure, mitral regurgitation

Q7. What is *pulsus bisferiens*?

A7. Pulsus fis feriens is

- A double – peaked arterial pulse, with both peaks in systole, and both peaks usually the same height (strength)
- Characterized by
  - Rapid upstroke
  - ↑ amplitude
  - Rapid downstroke
- Caused by
  - Aortic regurgitation
  - High output states
- The pulsus bisferiens may be heard as a
  - "pistol shot" femoral bruit
  - Duroziez' double murmur

Adapted from: Mangione S. *Hanley & Belfus* 2000, page 185.

Q8. What causes a *rapid arterial upstroke* when input and cardiac pulse pressure are normal?

A8.
- VSD, mitral regurgitation
- HOCM (hypertropic obstructive cardiomyopathy

A rapid arterial upstroke occurs with high output states (e.g. anemia, exercise, thyrotoxicosis, pregnancy, beriberi, Paget disease; AV fistulas

Q9. In which conditions may the pulse rate *in one arm differ* from that in the other?

A9. Usually, slowing of the pulse on one side occurs distal to the aneurymal sac. Thus, an aneurysm of the transverse or descending aortic arch causes a retardation of the left radial pulse. Also, the artery feels smaller and is more easily compresses than usual. An aneurysm of the ascending aorta or common carotid artery may result in similar changes in the right radial pulse.

Source: Baliga RR. *Saunders/Elsevier* 2007, page 94.

Q10. What is a "*Spike and dome bifid pulse*"?

A10.

- First peak from rapid early-systolic emptying of ventricle, then an obstruction, followed by another emptying (second peak).
- Association with severe HOCM

Source: Mangione S. *Hanley & Belfus* 2000, page 185.

Q11. What is "reversed *pulsus paradoxus*"?

A11.

- Pulsus paradoxus: inspiratory fall in systolic blood pressure (SBP) > 12 mm Hg (some authors say >10 mm Hg)
- Reversed pulsus paradoxus:
    - Expiratory fall in SBP>10 mm Hg
    - Caused by
        - HOCM
        - inspiration
        - acceleration of the sinus heart rate
        - intermittent inspiratory positive pressure breathing in L-CHF.

Source: Mangione S. *Hanley & Belfus* 2000, page 31.

Q12. About 98% of persons with pulsus paradoxus have cardiac tamponade. Your question: What do the *remainder* shave?

A12.
- Atrial septal defects
- Severe left ventricular dysfunction (especially with uremic pericarditis)
- Regional tamponade (tamponade affecting only one or two heart chambers, a complication of cardiac surgery)
- Severe hypotension
- Mechanical ventilation, the amount of pulsus paradoxus, correlates with the degree of the patient's auto-positive end-expiratory pressure (auto-PEEP) (a measure of expiratory difficulty in ventilated patients).
- Aortic regurgitation - BEWARE: with AR from type A aortic dissection, the hemopericardium may eliminate the pulsus paradoxus (PP), so the lack of PP in a person with dissection does not exclude tamponade.

Source: McGee SR. *Saunders/Elsevier* 2007, page 130.

Q13. What is the *difference* between pulsus alternans, pulsus bisferiens, and pulsus parvus?

A13.
- Pulsus alternans: strong-weak, strong-weak peripheral artery strength due to severe LV dysfunction.
- Pulsus bisferien's are palpable peaks in systole, with fast upstroke and downstroke, with high pulse amplitude.
  - Occurs in severe aortic regurgitation (AR), and may be associated with concurrent aortic stenosis (AR+AS)
  - Pulsus bisforien's once LV dydfunction occurs
- Pulsus parvus (hypokinetic pulse of the low

amplitude)

- Aortic stenosis
- Mitral stenosis
- Cardiomyopathy
- ↓ LV filling or contraction

## 23. Peripheral vascular disease (PVD)

Q1. In the context of PVD, what is the *Buerger test*?

A1. Blanching" upon raising legs and "rubor" on dependency

Q2. In the context of PVD, what is the *De Weese test*?

A2. Disappearance of palpable distal pulses after exercise

## 24.R/ LBBB

Q1. Distinguish between RBBB and LBBB, by listening to the *heart sounds*(!)

A1.
- RBBB: $A_2$-$P_2$ – when moving stethoscope from cardiac base to apex, the second component of $S_2$ disappears; associated with wide splitting of $S_2$.

- LBBB: $P_2$-$A_2$ – first component of $S_2$ becomes softer when moving stethoscope from the base to the apex of the heart ($A_2$ and not $P_2$ is heard at the apex).

## 25. Subacute bacterial endocarditis (SBE)

Q1. What is the most common *cause of death* in persons with SBE?

A1. CHF, secondary to
- o Perforation of a valve cusp
- o Rupture of a chorda tendinea

Q2. In the context of the patient with suspected SBE (subacute bacterial endocarditis), how do you different *Roth spots* from other types of red lesions of the retina?

A2. Red lesions of the retina are caused by
- o Microaneurysm
- o Blot an dot hemorrhages
- o Flame and splinter hemorrhages
- o Preretinal hemorrhages, including subhyaloid hemorrhages space
- o Roth spots are hemorrhages with a fibrinous centre which gives them a white spot with a red halo.
- o White- Centered hemorrhages are associated with
  - SBE
  - Diabetes
  - Intracranial hemorrhage
  - Leukemias
  - Various infectious processes

Adapted from: Mangione S. *Hanley & Belfus* 2000, page 99.

Q3. In the context of reddish lesions on the palms of the hands or soles of the feet, distinguish between *Janeway lesions* and *Osler's nodes*.

A3. Janeway lesions are small and non-tendon whereas, Osler's nodes are swollen, tender. Janeway lesions arise from septic emboli or sterile vasculitis in endocarditis (with or without bacteremia, gonococcal sepsis, or lupus (SLE).

## 26. Tricuspid regurgitation (TR)

Q1. What is the explanation for the murmur of TR (tricuspid regurgitation) not being auscultated *loudest* at the left lower sternal border or epigastric area?

A1.
- When the RV enlarges from TR and displaces the LV laterally and posteriorly, the murmur of TR will then be heard best at the right sternal border or apex
- If the person with TR has COPD and air trapping, the murmur will be heard over the free edge of the liver.

Source: Mangione S. *Hanley & Belfus* 2000, page 264.

Q2. In the context of inspiration and its effect on cardiac murmurs, what is the Rivera-Carvallo [RC] maneuver), and how does it differ from *Carvallo sign*?

A2.
- R-C maneuver
  - Inspiration cause a louder murmur across the pulmonic valve
- C. sign
  - Inspiration causes a louder pansystolic murmur of TR (tricuspid regurgitation, cluring or at the end of inspiration)
  - Carvallo sign has high specificity but only 61% sensitivity to distinguish TR from MR (mitral regurgitation, in which inspiration does not cause a louder murmur).

Source: Mangione S. *Hanley & Belfus* 2000, page 218 and 258.

## 27. Valsalva

Q1. During the strain phase of the Valsalva maneuver, there is increased intrathoracic pressure, which leads to a decrease in venous return and therefore a reduction of the blood volume moving into the LV. Thus, straining reduces the loudness of heart sounds and murmurs, because of the decrease in cross-valvular gradients. So what is the question?

What are the two *exceptions* to the Valsalva maneuver softening heart sounds/murmurs during the held phase?

A1.
- o HOCM (hypertrophic obstructive cardiomyopathy)
- o MVP (mitral valve prolapse)

Source: Mangione S. *Hanley & Belfus* 2000, page 257 and 268.

## 28. Vessels in the neck

Q1. Is the vessel in the neck the *jugular vein* (JV) or the *carotid artery* (CA).

A1.

| | JV | CA |
|---|---|---|
| o Inwards x,y waves | ✓ | No |
| o Upper level | ✓ | No |
| o Upper level falls with inspiration | ✓ | No |
| o Seen, better than felt | ✓ | No |
| o Felt, better than seen | No | ✓ |

Jugular Venous Pressure (JVP)

- 'a' ○ Atrial contraction
  - absent in AF
  - prominent in
    - PHT
    - PS
    - TS
- 'x' ○ Atrial relaxation
- 'y' ○ Tricuspid valve opens
- 'c' ○ Tricuspid valve closes
- 'v' ○ Venous blood returns to RA
  - ○ Not due to contraction of ventricle
  - ○ Often prominent in TR



Abbreviation: PHT, pulmonary hypertension; PS, pulmonary stenosis; TS, tricuspid stenosis; TR, tricuspid regurgitation; RA, right atrium.

Q2. In the context of the JVP, what is *Kussmaul sign*, and what are the *causes* of the Kussmaul sign being present?

A2.
- Kussmaul sign is a reversal of the usual fall in JVP with inspiration
- An increase in JVP with inspiration (Kussmaul sign) is present in
  - Constrictive pericarditis
  - Severe R-CHF

Q3. What are the performance characteristics of a "*carotid shudder*"?

A3. A palpable thrill on the slow stroke (pulsus tardis)
- Definition of carotid shudder
- Carotid shudder arises from the transmission of the murmurs of AS, AR, or AS plus AR to the artery.
- "... relatively specific but insensitive sign of aortic valvular disease"

Source: Mangione S. *Hanley & Belfus* 2000, page 186.

Q4. In which side of the neck is the carotid bruit best auscultated in the person with an iatrogenic *forearm AV* fistula prepared for hemodialysis?

A4. Louder carotid bruit on the same side as the AV fistula.

Q5. Atherosclerotic disease is common in persons with chronic renal failure (CRF). In the CRF patient with an AV *fistula* for hemodialysis, what sign, if present, favors the cause of the carotid bruit to be due to the *fistula* rather than being due to a carotid stenosis?

A5.An Associated subclavian bruit.

Q6. What is the *clinical significance* of auscultating a *carotid bruit*?

A6.

- Asymptomatic
  - Age 50, male
  - Preoperative
    - 3 x ↑ annual risk of CVA, TIA, death from coronary heart disease
    - ↑ risk of postoperative dysfunction and behavior problems (but <u>not</u> predictive of ↑ post-op risk of CVA)
- Symptomatic
    - ↑ risk of 70% to 99% stenosis ("high-grade" stenosis)

Q7. How can you assess central venous pressure (*CVP*) from the left internal jugular vein (IJV)?

A7. The right IJV more directly reflects right atrial pressure, and CVP measured on left side is higher than on the right side.

## Endocrinology

### 1. Adrenal glands

Q1. What is the *distinction* between Cushing disease, Cushing syndrome and pseudo-Cushing syndrome?

A1.
- Cushing disease is caused by pituitary adenoma, increased ACTH levels, and increased adrenal production of steroids

- Cushing syndrome is caused by increased steroids from any cause:
    - Steroids, including adrenocorticotropic hormone (ACTH)
    - Pituitary adenoma (Cushing disease)
    - Adrenal adenoma
    - Adrenal carcinoma
    - Ectopic ACTH (usually from small cell carcinoma of the lung)

- Pseudo-Cushing syndrome
    - Chronic alcoholics or depressed persons
    - ↑ urinary steroids, no diurnal variation in steroids, positive over-night dexamethasone test, all of which return to normal when causative factors abate

Source: Baliga RR. *Saunders/Elsevier* 2007, pages 386 and 387.

Q2. The prevalence of denial is of epidemic proportions in persons with increased body mass (aka "*obesity*"). When a patient claims "doctor, it's my glands", what endocrine causes do you consider?

A2.
- o Hypothyroidism
- o Hypogonadism
- o Cushing's syndrome
- o Insulinoma
- o Stein- Leventhal syndrome

Q3. In the same context, what is *Nelson syndrome*?

A3. o Bilateral adrenalectomy leading in 50% to increased ACTH levels, pituitary adenoma, hyperpigmentation

Source: Baliga RR. *Saunders/Elsevier* 2007, pages 386 and 387.

**2. Parathyroid**

Q1. On the basis of just the physical examination as well as the serum calcium (Ca) and phosphate ($PO_4$) concentrations, and their response to PTH, distinguish between the following three *variations of hypoparathyroidism*:

| A1. | Hypo-parathyroidism | Pseudo-hypo-parathyrodism* | Pseudo-pseudo-hypo-parathyroidism |
|---|---|---|---|
| Ca | ↓ | ↓ | N |
| $PO_4$ | ↑ | ↑ | N |
| Response to TSH | Yes | No | No |
| Skeletal changes | | Yes ** | Yes |

*conceptualize as "end-organ non-responsiveness
** Typical skeletal changes
- o Short neck
- o Short fingers
- o Less than 5 fingers

Q2. What are the *neurological changes* associated with hyperparathyroidism?

A2.
- Cataracts
- Papilloedema
- Basal ganglia defects
- Benign intracranial hypertension

Source: Burton J.L. *Churchill Livingstone* 1971, page 81.

Q3. Give 4 *radiological signs* for hyperparathyroidism.

A3.
- Subperiosteal erosions
  - Femoral necks
  - Fingers, middle phalanges
  - Fragmental cortex of phalanges
- Multiple bone cysts
  - May project from surface of affected bone
  - Often affects the jaw) osteitis fibrosa cystic)
  - Aka von Reckling harsen's disease
- Loss of lamina dura around teeth
- Punctuate translucencies of the skull ("mottling" or "pepper-pot skull")

Source: Davies IJT. *Lloyd-Luke (medical books) LTD* 1972, pages 222 and 223.

Q4. What are the effects of *renal osteodystrophy*?

A4.
- Secondary hyperparathyroidism
- Osteoporosis
- Osteomalacia

**3. Thyroid gland**

Q1. From the clinical examination, how might you suspect that you are dealing with hypothyroidism due to *pituitary failure*, rather than primary failure of the thyroid?

A1. Persons with hypopituitarism have

- Smooth skin
- Loss of body hair
- Long-term, there may be atrophy of the thyroid

Q2. Under what circumstances may a *bruit* be head over a carcinoma of the thyroid?

A2. When the uptake of radioactive iodine into the papillary or follicular carcinoma has been enhanced by increasing the blood supply to the thyroid with a drub such as carbimazole.

Q3. When you find a *midline mass*, what is the way on physical examination to distinguish between a thyroid lesion and a thyroglossal cyst?

A3. Both move on swallowing, but only the thyroglossal cyst moves when the tongue is protruded.

Q4. What is the way to demonstrate a *laryngocele*?

A4. A laryngocele may be demonstrated by performing the valsalva maneuver ("forced expiration against a closed glottis [bearing down], which increased intrathoracic and central nervous pressure, pushing on the diverticulum and making it more prominent in the area of the hyoid and thyroid cartilages.

Q5. Distinguish clubbing and bony enlargement from *thyroid acropachy* from pulmonary hypertrophic osteoarthropathy (*periostits*)

A5.
- Thyroid periostitis – hands and feet, asymptomatic
- Pulmonary hypertrophic osteoarthropathy – long bones

Source: Mangione S. *Hanley & Belfus* 2000, page 163.

Q6. Give some of the less important *eponyms* related to thyroid eye disease

A6.
- Infrequent blinking – Stellwag sign
- Tremor of gently closed eyelids – Rosenbach sign
- Difficulty in everting upper eyelid – Gifford sign
- Absence of wrinkling of forehead on sudden upward gaze – Joffroy sign
- Impaired convergence of the eyes following close accommodation – Möbius sign
- Weakness of at least one of the extraocular muscles – Ballet sign
- Paralysis of extraocular muscles – Jendrassik sign

Source: Baliga RR. *Saunders/Elsevier* 2007, page 36.

Q7. In the context of thyroid disease, what is the *Berry sign*?

A7. Berry's sign is the loss of the carotid pulse due to a thyroid malignancy causing enlargement of the thyroid to the point of blocking the carotid artery.

Q8. In the context of examining the thyroid gland, distinguish between the *Oliver sign*, *Cardarelli sign*, and *Campbell sign*.

A8.

- **Oliver sign**
  - "tracheal tug"
  - Downward displacement of the cricoids cartilage with each contraction of the ventricles
  - In a person with an aneurysm of the aortic arch each systolic ejection is transmitted by the dilated aortic arch onto the left bronchus, and from the left main bronchus to the trachea, pulling it downwards with each contraction of the ventricles.
- **Cardarelli sign**
  - When pressing on the thyroid cartilage to displace the thyroid to the left, a transverse pulsation is noted from the contact created between the left bronchus and the aorta, suggesting an aneurysm of the aortic arch.
- **Campbell sign**
  - When breathing in , the cartilage of the thyroid moves downwards (tracheal tug)
  - Associated with chronic obstructive pulmonary disease (COPD)
  - The degree of downward displacement ("tug") on the cartilage and therefore on the thyroid and the trachea
  - In COPD, there is strong contraction of the diaphragm, which pulls on the trachea during inspiration.

Q9. What is the usual cause of *unilateral proptosis*?

A9. Malignancy, not Grave disease (bilateral in 95%, thus unilateral in only 5%)

Q10. In the context of the eyebrows, what is the *Queen Anne sign*?

A10. Thinning of the hair of the eyebrows.

Q11. What conditions other than cosmetic practice and hypothyroidism are associated with thinning of *the eyebrows*?

A11.
- Systemic Lupus Erythematosis (SLE)
- Miscellaneous drugs and skin diseases

Q12. Stump the staff! How do you distinguish between thinning of the brows from SLE versus hypothyroidism?

A12. In hypothyroidism, it is the outer portion of the brow which is thinned.

Adapted from: Mangione S. *Hanley & Belfus* 2000, page 11.

Q13. Which signs of *Grave disease* are not due to the associated hyperthyroidism?

A13.
- Pretibial myxedema
- Exophthalmos

Q14. Which two functional thyroid disorders are associated with pretibial myxedema?

A14.
- Grave disease
- Hypothyroidism

Q15. In the patient with diffuse thyromegaly and unilateral proptosis, what are the causes of the *ophthalmopathy*?

A15. Although bilateral proptosis is the commonest cause of proptosis in adults, unilateral proptosis occurs in only 5% of Grave patients, so the correct answer is – lack for a cause of unilateral proptosis other than Grave disease.

Q16. What is *thyroid acropachy*, and how is it distinguished from a pulmonary etiology?

A16.

| | Acropachy thyroid | Pulmonary |
|---|---|---|
| o Painful periostitis | No | ✓ |
| o Long bones | No | ✓ |
| o Hands, feet | ✓ | No |

"Being happy doesn't mean that everything is perfect. It means that you've decided to look beyond the imperfections"

Unknown

# Gastroenterology

## *Mouth*

### 1. Gum Hypertrophy

Q1. Give 6 causes of *gum hypertrophy.*

A1.
- Gingivitis
    - from smoking
    - calculus
    - plaque
    - Vincent's angina (fusobacterial membranous tonsillitis)
- Drugs (Phenytoin)
- Pregnancy
- Scurvy (vitamin C deficiency: the gums become spongy, red, bleed easily and are swollen and irregular)
- Leukemia (usually monocytic)

Adapted from: Talley NJ, et al. *Maclennan & Petty Pty Limited* 2003, Table 5.6, page 161.

### 2. Pigmented lesions

Q1. Give 6 causes of *pigmented lesions* in the mouth, including tongue

A1.
- Drugs/Toxins
    - Heavy metals: lead or bismuth (blue-black line on the gingival margin), iron (hemochromatosis- blue-grey pigmentation of the hard palate)

- Drugs
  - Antimalarials
  - Oral contraceptive pill (brown or black areas of pigmentation anywhere in the mouth)

- Endocrine
  - Addison's disease (blotches of dark brown pigment anywhere in the mouth)
- Tumor
  - Malignant melanoma (raised, painless black lesions anywhere in the mouth)
- Genetic
  - Peutz- Jeghers syndrome (lips, buccal mucosa or palate)

Source: Talley NJ, et al. *Maclennan & Petty Pty Limited* 2003, Table 5.7, page 161.

### 3. Tongue, gum and Teeth Inspection

Q. Give 10 diagnoses which can be made from *inspection of the tongue, gums and teeth.*

A1.
- Magenta-colored tongue, angular stomatitis, cheilosis (cracked lips).
- Red side and tip of tongue (nicotinic acid deficiency)
- Depapillation glossitis (antibiotic therapy).
- Large tongue-myxedema, acromegaly, amyloid, Down syndrome
- Jaundice (frequently appears first and disappears last from frenulum of tongue)
- Scrotal tongue (normal or in Down syndrome)

- Geographical tongue-patchy reddish depapillation surrounded by “fur” (of no importance)
- Brown mottling of enamel (Fluorosis)
- Stippling of gums (Pb, bismuth poisoning)
- Furred tongue-fever (acute abdomen, uremia, cholemia)

Source: Mangione S. *Hanley & Belfus* 2000, page 122 and pages130-133.

Q2. Give 4 causes of an enlarged tongue (*macroglossia*).

A2.
- Acromegaly
- Hypothyroidism
- Amyloidosis
- Down syndrome

**4. Colored Mouth**

Q1. Give 6 lesions seen in the mouth, which are pigmented (not white)?

A1.
- Amalgam tattoo
- Peutz-Jeghers syndrome
- Smokers melanosis
- Hemochromatosis (15-25% of patients have a bluish-gray pigmentation of the hard palate with a lesser degree of pigmentation in the gingiva)
- Malignant melanoma (pigmented lesion with irregular borders, which may be palpable; often ulcerates)

- Black tongue, normal variant, associated with ingestion of iron tablets, bismuth, black liquorice.
- Addison's disease thus, the scattered melanotic spots
- Normal in African-Americans. This condition, termed "melanoplakia"

Source: Mangione S. *Hanley & Belfus* 2000, page 127.

## 5. White Spots in Mouth

Q1. What are the causes of *white spots* on the oral mucosa?

A1.
- Thickened oral mucosa
  - Broken tooth
  - Poorly fitting dentures
- Squamous cell carcinoma
- Infection
  - Candidiasis
  - Rubeola, echovirus, adenovirus, (cluster of ting white macules on buccal mucosa or first and second molars, known as Koplik's spots)
  - HIV - hairy leukoplakia on lateral aspects of tongue and buccal mucosa
- Leucoplakia is a term which was used in the past to imply a malignant lesion, but don't use this term because as you see from above, not all white lesions are malignant, just like not all Koplik's spots are caused by Rubella

Adapted from: Mangione S. *Hanley & Belfus* 2000, page 125.

***Esophagus***

## 1. GERD / NERD

Q1. In the person with heartburn but a normal EGD (esophagogastroduodenoscopy), what are the performance characteristics of the *Bernstein test*?

A1.
- Indication
  - Assess esophageal acid sensitivity in persons with NCCP or NERD.
  - Sensitivity 0-59%*
  - Specificity 59-94%

*Lack of association between symptoms induced by acid perfusion of esophagus compared with symptoms following spontaneous reflux in same individual, suggesting that heartburn following acid perfusion and spontaneous heartburn are induced by different stimuli.

Abbreviations: NCCP, non-cardiac chest pain; NERD, normal endoscopy reflux disease

Q2. When is a Virchow's node *not a Virchow's node*?

A2
- Virchow's node is a left supraclavicular node fro metastasis from a gastric cancer
- When a left supraventricular node is metastatic from cancer of the esophagus, or an ipsilateral breast (L) or lung cancer, it is called a Troisier's node (!!)

"Goals allow you to control the direction of change in your favor."

Brian Tracy

## 2. Achalasia

Q1. Give 2 causes of postsurgical pseudoachalasia (secondary achalasia).

A1.

| | |
|---|---|
| o After fundoplication | - Motility changes may be similar<br>- Amyl nitrate markedly reduces LES in primary than in postsurgical achalasia<br>- Ensure that postfundoplication dysphagia and possibly associated achalasia-like symptoms are not due to a paraesophageal hernia. |
| o After laproscopic adjustable gastric banding (GB, bariatric surgery) | - 14% of LAGB have postoperative dilation of esophagus > 3.5 cm<br>- Mechanism unknown<br>- Usually this form of secondary achalasia resolves with removal of the gastric band |

Q2. On high resolution esophageal manometry, define the three esophageal segments, and give the method of calculation and the use of the CFV (contractile front velocity) for defining an esophageal spastic contraction.

A2.
- o There is one proximal esophageal body segment ($S_1$), and the three distal esophageal segments ($S_2$, $S_3$, and $S_4$)

- The pressure minimum in the transition zone at the lower portion of the upper third of the esophagus represents $S_1$, resulting from skeletal muscle
- The lower two thirds of the esophageal body represents the distal esophageal segment formed from smooth muscle.
- Within the distal esophageal segment there are three pressure peaks, $S_2$, $S_3$, and $S_4$
- Connect the proximal margin of $S_2$ and the distal margin of $S_3$
- Calculate the slope of the line connecting the 30 cm Hg isobaric contour (IBC) line

Q3. Using HREP manometry terms, distinguish between the three subtypes of achalasia (both a peristalsis and impaired deglutitive EGJ relaxation are needed to diagnose achalasia).

| Subtypes of achalasia | Pressurization of esophageal body | IRP (mm Hg) | CFV (cm / sec) | Overall treatment response |
|---|---|---|---|---|
| I classical (20%) | - | ≥ 15 | < 8 | 56% |
| II compression (50%) (panesophageal)* | + | ≥ 15 | > IRP** | 96% |
| III spastic (30%) | - | ≥ 15 | > 8 | 29% |

- Highly predictive of good response to treatment

* With compartmentalized esophageal pressurization, the 30 cm long and the 50 cm long IBC (isobaric

contour) lines are not parallel to each other

- In type II, there is no esophageal dilation, as there is with type III

** - In penesophageal compression achalasia, the ↑ IRP (integrated relaxation pressure, i.e., the causes the pressure in the body of the esophagus to be compartmentalized with high intrabolus pressure developing between the "contractile front of the distal esophageal contraction and the EGJ……" (Feldman M., et al. *Saunders/Elsevier 2010*, page 696).

- As a result of this intrabolus pressure compartmentalization, the slope of the 30 cm isobar contour line no longer represents the CFV, so "…the algorithm for computing CFV defaults to computing the slope of an isobaric contour line of magnitude greater than the EGJ relaxation pressure….so as to consistently represent the timing of the luminal closure.

Q4. Achalasia may be associated with degenerative neurological disorders, such as Parkinson disease. The typical pathophysiological defect seen in biopsies of the esophagus of patients with achalasia is reduced (inhibitory) ganglion cells.

In persons with achalasia associated with *Parkinsonism*, what are the characteristics of the *degenerating* esophageal ganglion cells?

A4. The degenerating ganglion cells in persons with achalasia associated with Parkinsion disease show intracytocytoplasmic hyaline or spherical eosinophilic inclusions. These intracytoplasmic hyaline or spherical eosinophilic inclusions are called "Lewy bodies".

Q5. It is thought that the major pathophysiological defect in *achalasia* in dysfunction / loss of inhibitory ganglion nerve (IGN).

On the basis of the typical manometric changes in achalasia, give two pieces of evidence that this IGN dysfunction theory is correct.

A5.
- o Important in "deglutitive inhibition", i.e., swallow-associated LES, relaxation
- o This impaired deglutitive inhibition leads to failure of relaxation of LES with swallowing which occurs in achalasia
- o Important in "sequenced propagation" of esophageal peristalsis
  - This impaired sequence propagation leads to a peristalsis of smooth muscle of body of esophagus.

Q6. What is the normal effect of *CCK* on esophageal muscle, and what is its effect in achalasia.

A6. Normal - CCK → ↓ LES (i.e., ↑ LES contraction)
Achalasia - CCK paradoxically ↑ LES pressure (i.e. ↓ LES relaxation)
- this may explain why LES pressure may be increased in 60% of persons with achalasia

Q7. Pulmonary aspiration from food / fluid trapped in the esophagus from impaired relaxation of the LES is common in achalasia. Give the significance of the development of *stridor* (large airway compromise) in achalasia.

A7. With failure of relaxation of the LES and a peristalsis in achalasia, the esophagus may dilate sufficient to compress the trachea

Q8. Patients with achalasia may experience regurgitation of food on fluid as the result of food and fluid not passing into the stomach. But when "*heartburn*" develop in an achalasia patient, what is the mechanism?

A8.
- Myotomy treatment used for or smooth muscle relaxing drugs
- Retained food in esophagus fermented to acidic short chain fatty acids (e.g., acetic, butyric, proprionic acids)

Q9. Chest pain distinct from heartburn-like retrosternal burning discomfort may occur in as many as two thirds of achalasia patients. What is the *mechanism* of this pain?

A9.
- Spasm of longitudinal smooth muscle of esophagus
- Dilation of esophagus (megaesophagus)

Q10. Which manometric feature helps to differentiate spastic achalasia from distal DES (diffuse esophageal spasm)?

A10. Both DES and spastic achalasia may have non-peristaltic esophageal wave in the body of the esophagus, but only achalasia shows impaired relaxation of LES.

Q11. Why must the patient with *oropharyngeal dysphagia* always be assessed for a possible esophageal disease / disorder?

A11. The localization of the site esophageal disease is poor; half of patients with a disease in the lower esophagus may experience their symptom in the area of the upper esophagus, so that symptoms perceived to arise from the upper esophagus may in fact be from the upper of the lower esophagus.

Q12. Give 4 features on history which help to determine if the feeling of a lump in the throat represents *globus*, rather than dysphagia.

A12. Globus

- o Present between meals, not with swallowing food as with dysphagia
- o Swallowing food/ liquids makes globus better, not worse
- o Emotional stress makes globus worse
- o Frequently associated psychiatric and somatization disorders

## 3. Dyspepsia

Q1. What is the mechanism of *cold – induced* esophageal pain?

A1. Esophageal spasm. Nope – you're back in the last century!. Cold induced esophageal pain results from distention of the esophagus. In fact, cold produces lack of esophageal peristalsis, resulting in dilation of the esophagus.

Q2. A simple question: *define* "heartburn".

A2. "A burning feeling rising from the stomach or lower chest up toward the neck" (www.expertconsult.com)

Q3. What is the *difference* between "uninvestigated dyspepsia" and "functional dyspepsia".

A3.
- o Uninvestigated dyspepsia" is pain a discomfort with upper abdomen, thought to be due to a disorder in the upper GI tract, "in persons in whom no diagnostic investigations have been performed and in when a specific diagnosis that explains the dyspeptic symptoms has not been determined"
- o "functional dyspepsia" is dyspepsia occurring in a person who has had an EGD (esophagogastroduodenoscopy), and the EGD is normal.

Q4. Dyspepsia is a symptom complex, with large heterogeneity of symptoms. There are a number of pathophysiological changes seen in persons with functional dyspepsia. The Rome criteria are respected as definitions for and guidance of the management of translucence GI disorders. The Rome III committee recommended that functional dyspepsia be considered as two subgroups:

- PDS (meal – related dyspeptic symptoms)
- EPS (meal – unrelated dyspeptic symptoms)

Give the validity use of these terms, PDS and EPS, in persons with functional dyspepsia.

A4. The validity of this classification and distinction is not evidence – based.

## 4. Esophageal bolus obstruction

- Esophageal Foreign Bodies

Incidence of Esophageal food bolus impaction, $16/10^5$ per year

Q1. A patient with an esophageal food-associated obstruction is given glucagon. What is the success rate of glucagon, what is its mechanism of action, and why is EGD still necessary if the food *bolus* passes?

A1.
- Success rate of glucagon ~ 50%
- Relaxation of LES pressure using glucagon ~50%
- Associated esophageal pathology, 75%
    - Peptic stricture
    - Schatzki's ring
    - Eosinophilic esophagitis

**5. Gastroenteropathy**

Q1. Give the laboratory features of *allergic gastroenteropathy*.

A1.
- ↓ serum
  - Albumin and total protein
  - Immunoglobins
  - Transferrin
  - ↑ eosinophils in lamina propria of affected GI tissues
  - Stool samples contain Charcot-Leyden crystals

**6. Lower esophageal sphincter relaxation**

Q1. Give 4 signals which alter the lower esophageal sphincter relaxation (LESR)

A1.
- ↑ TLESR
  - NO (nitric oxide)
  - CCK (cholecystokinin), acting through the CCK-A receptors
  - Muscarinic receptors
- ↓ TLESR
  - $GABA_s$ (γ-aminobutyric acid, or γ aminobutyric acid agonists)

"Happiness always sneaks in a door you did not think was open"

Anonymous

Q2. Give the signaling stimuli, sensory endings, different nerves and ganglia which modulate *esophageal sensation*

| Signaling (stimuli) | Sensory endings | Afferent nerves | Ganglia |
|---|---|---|---|
| - Mechanical<br>- Chemical<br>- Thermal<br>- Electrical | - IGLEs<br>▪ Tension sensitive<br>- IMAs<br>▪ Stretch sensitive<br>- Respond to 5-HT, ATP, bile | - Vagal<br>▪ Upper 1/3 – superior laryngeal nerve<br>▪ Lower 2/3 plus LES – branches of vagus<br>- Spincal<br>▪ Thoracic splanchnic<br>▪ mGlaR5 (metabotropic glutamate receptor) antagonists inhibit TLESR | - Jugular<br>- Nodose<br>- Cervical of thoracic dorsal root |

Abbreviations:

- IGLEs
  - Intraganglionic laminar [free nerve] endings in the myenteric ganglia
  - In a "….laminar structure that encapsulates the myenteric ganglia" (Feldman M., et al. *Saunders/Elsevier* 2010, page 686).
  - Predominanatly tension-sensitive afferents
  - IGLEs in the proximal stomach mediate TLESR (IGLEs → medulla → vagal efferents and phrenic nerves)
- IMAs
  - Intramuscular arrays in the muscularis propria,
  - Mostly in the LES
  - Mostly stretch-sensitive

- Forming a network with ICCs (interstitial cells of the Cajal)
- ASICs
  - GI-acid sensing ion channels involved in mechanotransduction and response to acid
  - Releases inflammatory substances and neuropeptides
- TRPV1
  - Transient receptor potential vanilloid – 1
- 5-HT, 5-hydroxytryptamine
- ATP, adenosine triphosphate
- Dilated (> 1.69 mm) (intercellular spaces) is the earliest sign of damage to the esophageal epithelial cells. The resulting ↑ paracellular permeability to hydrochloric acid, pepsin and bile acids stimulates receptors for the sensory neurons in the intercellular space, resulting in “heartburn”.
- Gastropharyngeal reflux symptom severity falls after age 31 to 40 years, but the risk of associated esophagitis associated with symptoms necrosis.

Feldman M., et al. *Saunders/Elsevier* 2010, page 708.

## 7. Comparison of LES vs TLESR

Q1. About 10% of reflex episodes in health persons occurring when there is swallow-associated LESR, and the rest occur when there is incomplete peristalsis. Give 2 reasons why reflux during swallowing-induced LESR is so uncommon.

A1.
- LESR lasts only 5 to 10 seconds, so there is little time for reflux to occur.
- The crural diaphragm does not relax during swallowing, thereby acting as a barrier to reflux
- The approaching peristaltic waves push any refluxate body into the stomach.

Q2. Give 6 means by which the presence of a sliding esophageal hiatus hernia (HH) contributes to GERD.

A2.
- o In the presence of a HH, the EGJ has a lower compliance, so that the EGJ may open at pressure lower than the intragastric pressure.
- o Esophagitis associated with an HH may release mediators which ↓ LESP.
- o As LESP falls, there is an increased likelihood of reflux.
- o The presence of the HH reduces the support of the crural diaphragm.
- o Loss of the intra-abdominal high pressure zone
  - – Proximal displacement of the LES, or
  - – Shortening of the esophagus
- o ↓ straining-associated ↑ LESP
- o ↑ gastric-distention associated ↑ TLESRs
- o ↓ esophageal acid clearance
- o HH is commonly associated with esophagitis (> 50%)
- o HH increases risk of esophagitis (not just GER)

Q3. Give the endoscopic definition of a *non-reducible* esophageal hernia.

A3.
- o A non-reducible hiatus hernia is one in which ".... The gastric rugal folds remain above the diaphragm between swallows" (Feldman M., et al. *Saunders/Elsevier* 2010, page 710)

Q4. Over half of GERD patients have sleep disturbances. Give the changes in esophageal function during *sleep*.

A4. ○ During sleep in the supine position, there is

- ↓ effect of gravity
- ↓ salination
- ↓ esophageal secondary peristalsis

Q5. The contents of the esophageal lumen are buffered by the alkaline, $HCO_3^-$ rich submucosal glands of the esophagus. Give the chemicals which buffer the *intracellular pH* of the esophagus.

A5. ○ The intracellular contents of the squamous mucosa of the esophagus are buffered by

- $HCO_3^-$
- Phosphates
- Protein

Q6. TRPV1 (*vanilloid receptor 1*) is expressed on sensory neurons of the esophagus; what is its function.

A6. ○ TRPV1 is activated by

- Chemicals ($H^+$, bile acids)
- Heat
- Distention

○ As such, TRPV1 may mediate the sensation, reported by patients as "heartburn"

○ It is unknown why only ~ 20% of GE reflux episodes are associated with symptoms

Q7. Give the earliest *cellular marker* of GERD, and its dimensions.

A7.
- o The normal intercellular spaces in the esophagus of normal persons is < 1.69 μm.
- o Dilation beyond this value occurs by unknown mechanisms, and is the earliest sign of mucosal damage from $H^+$, pepsin, and bile acids

Q8. In the context of GERD, what is the "*acid pocket*"?

A8.
- o At the LES, extending from the lower esophagus into the cardia, there is an acid pocket, which is not neutralized by the presence of food buffering the gastric acidity.
- o In the LES area, the pH < 4 for about one quarter of the 24 hour day (a reflux episode is define as pH drop of < 4.
- o Physiological reflux is limited to pH < 4 for 5.5% of the 24 hour day.
- o This increased acid exposure may predispose to damage from GE reflux at this area.
- o This has a sensitivity for esophagitis of 77% to 100%, and specificity of 85% to 100%.

Q9. You suspect that your patient's hoarseness is due to GERD. An EHT consultation agrees the patient has "*reflux laryngitis*". Give the laryngoscopic findings which would expect to have been seen.

A9.
- o Reflux laryngitis is characterized endoscopically as
  - Redness of the medial arytenoid walls, in the interarytenoid areas
  - Red streaks on the posterior third of the vocal cord folds

Q10. Compare the *performance characteristics* of an empirical PPI trial for GERD versus NCPP (non-cardiac chest pain).

A10.
- For GERD, the PPI test represents standard dose PPI bid for 2 weeks, with 50% decrease in heartburn.
- For NCCP, the PPI test represents twice normal PPI dose in the AM and night time single standard dose (e.g. omeprazole 40 mg in AM and 20 mg pm)

| | GERD | NCCP |
|---|---|---|
| o Sensitivity | 68% to 83% | 78% |

- RR of NCCP with PPIs versus placebo: 0.54 (NNT, 3)

Q11. Over half of persons with typical GERD symptoms have a normal EGD. These patients are said to have (normal endoscopy reflux disease, non-erosive reflux disease, aka *functional dyspepsia*). Give the role of esophageal pH testing in the *subclassification* of the 3 types of NERD.

A11.

| Findings | Types 1 | 2 | 3 |
|---|---|---|---|
| o Abnormal esophageal pH testing | + | - | - |
| o Response to PPI: correlation between symptoms and episodes of reflux | + | + | - |

Q12. From the position of narrowing of the esophagus (*stricture*) seen on a barium esophagogram, give the likely cause.

A12.
- Mid – esophagus - Barrette epithelium-associated adenocarcinoma
- Lower esophagus - Schatzki ring

Q13. Give the role of surgery in *Zenker diverticulum.*

A13. Over 80% of patient with a hypopharyngeal (Zenker) diverticulum and cricopharyngeal bar respond to diverticulectomy plus myotomy; neither of these is recommended by itself, except possibly simple myotomy for a small diverticulum.

Feldman M, et al. *Saunders/Elsevier* 2010, page 708.

Q14. In the patient with symptoms of GERD, many treatment algorithms emphasize the importance of numerous "life-style-changes". Give the *life style changes* for which there is demonstrated efficacy in GERD.

A14. While the results from life-style changes may vary from one patient to another with symptoms of GERD, appropriately designed studies have provided evidence for benefit only for

- Elevation of the head of the bed
- Weight loss (if ↑ BMI)
- Lying down in the left lateral decubitus position space
- *Note that while the evidence for benefit from smoking cessation in GERD is not strong, physicians with often take the opportunity to advise GERD patients of the overall benefits of stopping the smoke.

Q15. In the context of ↑ TLESRs (transients lower esophageal sphincter relaxation) in persons with GERD, name four classes of drugs that reduce TLESRs.

A15. ↓ TLESRs may be achieved with

- Agonists $GABA_B$ (γ-amino butyric acid)
- CCK-1 receptor antagonists (CCKA)
- Anticholinergics (atropine)
- NO (nitric oxide) synthase inhibitors
- Morphine

Q16. Obesity is associated with an increased risk of GERD, BE and esophageal adenocarcinoma (ECa). Name 3 *peptides* which may be linked to this association.

A16.

- Obesity is associated with an ↑ risk of GERD, BE and Eca by way of
  - ↑ IGF-1 (insulin-like growth factor 1) (proliferative peptide)
  - ↑ leptin
  - ↓ adiponectin (anti-proliferative effect of adiponectin)

Q17. There is progressively increased genetic instability of the normal esophageal mucosa progresses from metaplasia to dysplasia, and from dysplasia to esophageal adenocarcinoma.

Give 5 *genetic and epigenetic* alterations that endow the [esophageal squamous] cells with the physiological attributes of malignancy (Feldman M., et al. *Saunders/Elsevier* 2010, page 729), including the mediators associated with each alteration.

A17.

- Metaplasia

| | |
|---|---|
| o Self-sufficiency growth signals | – ↑ oncogenes (cyclin D1)<br>– ↑ growth factors (TGF-α), EGFR [epidermal growth factor receptor] |
| o ↓ sensitivity to anti-growth signals | – ↓ activation of tumor suppressor genes ($TP_{53}$, $TP_{16}$) |
| o ↑ angiogenesis<br>o ↑ aneuploidy<br>o ↑ abnormal cellular DNA content | – ↑ VEGF (vascular endothelial growth factor) |

➢ Dysplasia

| | |
|---|---|
| o Evasion of apoptosis | – ↓ activation of $TP_{53}$ |
| o ↑ replicative potential | – ↑ activation of telomerase, ↑ telomeres for cell division |
| o Tissue invasion and metastasis | – ↓ cell adhesion (↓ cadherins, ↓ catenins)<br>– ↑ extracellular matrix degeneration – (↑ MMPs [matrix metalloproteases] |

➢ Adenocarcinoma

| | |
|---|---|
| o Self-sufficiency in growth signals | – ↑ oncogene (K-Ras) |
| o self-sufficiency in growth signals | – ↑ oncogenes |

*Note that at least 10% of tissue with HGD (high grade dysplasia) will already contain in situ cancer

Adapted from: Feldman M, et al. *Saunders/Elsevier* 2010, page 729.

## 8. Epiphrenic diverticulum (ED)

Q1. What is the rational of performing *myotomy plus fundoplication* in persons with an ED?

A1. ED may occur as a complication of bariatric surgery, but 80% of ED is associated with a motility disorder of the esophagus. Thus, the myotomy needs to be done at the time of the resection of the ED to reduce the high risk of recurrence. With the myotomy, there is risk of post-resection GERD, so a non-destructing fundoplication is performed.

## 9. Esophageal Intramural Pseudodiverticular (EIP)

Q1. Define *EIP*, and list 4 of its complications.

A1. EIP are abnormally dilated ducts of the esophageal submucosal glands, leading to

- Periductal inflammation and fibrosis
- Strictures
- Communication between adjacent pseudodiverticula
- Ulceration, hemorrhage
- Perforation → mediastinitis
- Misdiagnosis of esophageal cancer

"Be helpful. When you see a person without a smile, give them yours"

Zig Ziglar.

## 10. Esophageal pressure

Q1. In the context of HREPT (high resolution esophageal pressure topography), define DCI (*distal contractile integrity*), and give two examples of its use.

A1.
- o Definition: "The DCI integrates the length, vigor and persistence of the two subsegments of the distal esophageal segment contraction" (Feldman M., et al. *Saunders/Elsevier* 2010, page 697).
- o Nutcracker esophagus (by conventional manometry, pressure waves of esophageal body > 180 mm Hg)
  - DCI > 5000 mm Hg.s.cm
- o "Spastic nutcracker" pattern
  - DCI > 8000 mm Hg.s.cm
- o Hypertensive LES

Q2. Using HREPT, give the three components which are measured and used to create the *Chicago classification* of esophageal motility disorders (see Feldman M., et al. *Saunders/Elsevier* 2010, Table 42.2, page 699).

A2.
- o IRP (integrated relaxation pressure, EGJ deglutitive relaxation)
- o CFV (contraction front velocity)
- o DCI (distal contractile interval)

## 11. Barrett epithelium

Q1. BE (Barrett epithelium) occurs in about one in ten persons with GERD. Give the criteria for the description of BE taking into account current controversies.

- Prague CM criteria
  - C, circumference
  - M, maximum extent (length)
- Long segment BE seen in 3% to 5% of GERD patients 10% to 20% short segment BE

A1.
- Country
  - USA
    - Endoscopic abnormality
    - "long" (> 3 cm) versus "short" (< 3 cm) segment

*Note: 5% of adults with non-GERD symptoms have BE

  - Europe
    - Biopsy abnormality (columnar epithelium, with goblet cells)

*Note: Dysplastic tissue may be patchy, and may appear normal on endoscopy)

- Biopsy
  - Metaplasia
    - intestinal metaplasia at the GE junction
    - metaplasia of gastric cardiac-type epithelium

Q2. Define "dysplasia", and give 5 changes in tissue *architecture* and cell *morphology* which are seen in this condition.

A2. The histological changes of dysplasia include:

- Architecture
  - Disorganized villiform surfaces
  - Crowded tubules
- Cell nucleus
  - Large nucleus
  - Pleomorphic hyperchromatic
  - Stratified
  - Atypical mitoses
- Cell cytoplasm
  - Loss of maturation

Q3. Give the approximate risk of BE metaplasia *progressing* to LGD (low grade dysplasia), HGD (high grade dysplasia), or ECa (esophageal adenocarcinoma) each year.

A3. BE metaplasia LCD HGD ECa

o---------------------------------→0.5%/year, or lower

o----------→ 4.3%/year

o-------------------→ 0.9%/year

o----→4% to 6% /year

o---------------------------------------------------→ 0.12% / year

Q4. In symptomatic patients with GERD or BE, elimination of symptoms does not mean that the gastric % pH < 4 is less than 4% to 5%, or that the esophagitis has resolves. What is the physiological explanation for this disconnect?

A4. The data on PPI gastric acid suppression and targeting 24 hr pH < 4 to < 5% is for gastric and not for esophageal pH may be low (↑ $H^+$). Thus, the use of gastric pH as a surrogate marker for esophageal pH must be challenged.

Q5. Some authorities recommend endoscopic surveillance for BE, and discourage anti-reflux surgery for the prevention of development of esophageal adenocarcinoma. While EMR (endoscopic mucosal resection does provide a pathological specimen" …….to judge the depth of neoplastic invasion and the completeness of the ablation" (Feldman M., et al. *Saunders/Elsevier* 2010, page 731), this "suck and cut" or "band and snare" approach does have a significant risk of recurrent or metachronous cancer. Ablation methods for BE do not provide tissue samples for pathological assessment, and there is the risk that the ablation treatment may leave metaplastic tissue "buried" under healing squamous mucosa which looks endoscopically normal.

Give the risk of *recurrent or metachronous* esophageal adenocarcinoma in BE patients treated with these two different modalities.

A5.

- The risk of developing esophageal adenocarcinoma after therapy for BE
  - PPI alone, 29%
  - PPI plus PDT (photodynamic therapy), 15% to 21% in 5 years
  - EMR, 11% in 37 months, 21% in 5 years
- Consider ASA plus PPI for the prevention or ↓ recurrent cancers
- If BE extends to a large portion of the circumference of the esophagus, perform EMR over several sessions in order to ↓ risk of formation of stricture.

## 12. Mallory Weiss Tear

Q1. The MW (Mallory-Weiss) syndrome arises from a tear in the esophagus, usually within 2 cm of the EGJ (esophagogastric junction), along the lesser curve of the cordia. The bleeding arising from the tear is proceeded by vomiting in about two thirds of patients.

Give *the mechanism* of the MW syndrome or tear.

A1. The MW tear is thought to arise from ".......shearing forces on the gastroesophageal junction and proximal stomach as it herniates through the diaphragm because of high intra-abdominal pressure due to forceful vomiting" (Feldman M., et al. *Saunders/Elsevier* 2010, page 740).

## 13. Infections

Q1. In the context of the immune-suppressed patient in the ICU who develop dysphagia and retrosternal pain, define the "*black esophagus*".

A1.
- The "black esophagus" represents the endoscopic finding of acute esophageal necrosis
- This may arise from esophageal ischemia, or infections such as candidiasis or HSV.

Q2. A 60 year old patient with dyspepsia has EGD showing multiple *white patches*.

Give ways to distinguish between candidiasis versus glycogenic acanthosis.

A2.

| Features | Candidiasis | Glycogenic acanthosis |
|---|---|---|
| ➢ History, immunosuppression | +/- | - |
| ➢ White patches wash away with EGD water infusion | + | - |
| ➢ Brushing for, cytology hyphaeon | + | - |
| ➢ Biopsy | Hyphae | Large squamous cells because of ↑ glycogen in cytoplasm |

Q3. Esophageal candidiasis is common in persons who are profoundly immune suppressed (e.g. HIV/AIDS, or post-transplantation). Give 7 additional conditions predisposing the patient to *candida esophagitis*.

A3. Conditions which predispose to the development of esophageal candidiasis include

- Esophageal stasis
  - Scleroderma
  - Achalasia
  - Stricture
  - Intramural pseudodiverticulosis
  - Eosinophilic esophagitis (possibly from treatment with topical steroids)

| | |
|---|---|
| ➢ Medications | o PPIs<br>o Topical steroids |
| ➢ Immune-suppression | o Old age<br>o Diabetes<br>o Alcoholism |

Q4. HPV (human papillomavirus) is a DNA virus which infects squamous epithelium of normal, immune competent persons. HPV infection is often asymptomatic. Give the endoscopic findings of *HPV esophagitis*.

A4. Because HPV is often asymptomatic, the diagnosis may be missed. When EGD is performed, the following endoscopic changes are characteristic:

- o Red macules
- o White patches
- o Nodules
- o Frond-like lesions
- o Associated esophageal squamous cell cancer in patients with APECED (autoimmune polyendocrinopathy-candidiasis-ectodermal dystrophy)

Q5. An immune suppressed patient with dyspepsia and odynophagia is found to have EGD. Give the endoscopic and biopsy changes which differentiate *CMV* versus *HSV esophagitis*.

A6.

| | CMV | HSV |
|---|---|---|
| ➢ Ulcers | ○ A few long, large, deep, serpiginous ulcers with undermined edges | ○ Numerous small, round, superficial "ulcer-like" ulcers |
| ➢ Location | ○ Mid and distal third | ○ Any part of esophagus |
| ➢ Biopsy | ○ Center of lesion<br>○ "Owl's eyes" inclusion bodies | ○ Edge of lesion<br>○ Nuclei, "ground glass"<br>○ Multinucleated giant cells<br>○ Eosinophilic "Cowdry bodies" |

Adapted from: Spiegel, BMR, et al. *Slack Incorporated* 2011, Table 147.1, page 180.

## 14. Esophageal Varices

Q1
- The risk of any patient with compensated cirrhosis having EV (esophageal varices) is high (50%),
- The risk of these EV bleeding is high (30% in next 2 years), and
- The risk of dying from this first EV bleeding is high (20%);
- It is important to identify all those cirrhotic patients who might have EV and therefore would benefit from EVBL (esophageal variceal band ligation).

If we were to accept that it is not cost-effective to perform EGD on all compensated cirrhotic to determine if EV are present, then indicate what *factors predict the presence of EV* in a patient with cirrhosis (↑ HVPG > 12 mm Hg), and which thereby be used to increase the pretest probability of finding EV on EGD.

A1.

- o Physical examination
  - – Splenomegaly
- o Laboratory
  - – Platelets < 88,000 / mL
  - – ↑ INR
- o Diagnostic imaging (abdominal ultrasound)
  - – Portal vein diameter > 13 mm

Abbreviations: EGD, esophagastroduodenoscopy; HVPG, hepatic vein pressure gradient

Q2. Give the pathophysiological basis for EVBL being superior to *β-blockers* for primary (before first EV bleed) or secondary (after first EV bleed) prophylaxis of EV (esophageal variceal) bleeding (EVB).

A2.

- ➢ B-blockers
  - o The risk of EVB is related to the HVPG
  - o The threshold for EVB is HVPG > 12 mm Hg
  - o B-blocker (BB) dosage is targeted to ↓ HVPG < 12 mm Hg, but it is not routinely possible to have HVPG measurements.
  - o Surrogate markers for BB ↓ HVPG < 12 mm Hg include
    - – ↓ HR to 55-60 bpm
    - – ↓ SBP by 25%
  - o Even with ↓ HR / ↓ SBP to these targets, the HVPG may still be > 12 mm Hg
  - o Also, the BB dosage may cause adverse effects and dose-escalation may need to be stopped before these HR / SBP endpoints are reached.
  - o Compliance with taking BB may be an issue

if there HR / SBP endpoints are reached

- Risk reduction for EVB with BB, only 50%

- EVBL (endoscopic variceal band ligation)
  - Risk reduction, 66%
  - Less compliance issue
  - May still provide some benefit, even when HVPG > 12 mm Hg

Q3. Varices may appear in the esophagus, at the junction of the esophagus and stomach (junctional varices), or as isolated gastric fundic varices. Fundic varices may occur in association with esophageal or junctional varices, when there is portal hypertension. When there are isolated *fundic varices*, the HVPG (hepatic venous pressure gradient) is normal (< 12 mm Hg).

Give the anatomical basis for isolated fundic varices.

A3.
- The splenic vein joins the superior mesenteric vein to form the portal vein (PV).
- The esophageal vein (EV) comes from the PV, so any obstruction which is proximal to the take-off of the EV from the PV causes left-sided portal hypertension, without esophageal or junctional varices.
- Thrombosis of the splenic vein leads to congestion of spleen and distention of the short gastric veins (SGV).
- Distention of the SGV leading from the spleen to the gastric fundus will cause isolated gastric fundal varices.
- The isolated gastric fundal varices.

Q4. The usual treatment of *isolated gastric fundal varices* arising from splenic vein thrombosis (SVT) is splenectomy.

Give the anatomical circumstances when a splenectomy will not be therapeutically successful to treat SVT and its associated left-sided portal hypertension.

A4. Splenectomy for SVT would not be useful to treat left-sided portal hypertension if thrombosis of the splenic veins were also associated with thrombosis of the inferior and/or superior mesenteric veins.

Q5. In a pregnant woman with cirrhosis, what are the risks of a *splenic artery aneurysm* (SAA)

A5..
- Risk of rupture, 5%
- Mortality rate in
  - Mother, 75%
  - Fetus, 90%
- Risk of rupture increases when SAA > 2 cm

Q6. In pregnancy, the portal pressure increases because of the physiological increase in plasma volume. In a pregnant woman with cirrhosis, give the *risk of variceal bleeding*.

A6.
- The risk of bleeding from esophageal varices during pregnancy depends on their size:
  - Small varices, 25%
  - Large varices, 75%

Q7. In a pregnant cirrhotic woman, there is a high risk of bleeding. There are no trials of the efficacy or safety of EVC (esophageal variceal ligation) in pregnant cirrhotic patients. Beta-blockade is useful for primary and secondary prophylaxis of esophageal variceal bleeding in non-pregnant cirrhotic, and beta-blockers are FDA pregnancy class C.

Give the reason why beta-blockers should not be used in the pregnant woman with cirrhosis.

A7.
- It is true that β-blockers are FDA pregnancy class C in $T_1$ (the first trimester of pregnancy), but in $T_2$ and $T_3$, β-blockers are FDA pregnancy class D.
- This class D rating in the second and third trimester is due to their adverse effect on the fetus at that time, due to fetal
  - Growth retardation
  - Bradycardia

**15. Hamartoma**

Q1. Define "*hamartoma*".

A1. Hamartomas are "....benign developmental tumors consisting of disorganized and excessive focal growth of the mature normal cells" (Feldman M., et al. *Saunders/Elsevier* 2010, page 769).

Give the therapeutic modalities available for *early esophageal cancers*.

- Endoscopic mucosal / submucosal resection (EMR / ESR). For early ECa)
  - Polypectomy snare
  - Lift-and-cut, with double channel endoscope
  - Band-and-cut
  - Cap assisted
  - Space

- EMR plus EAT (endoscopic ablative therapy)
  - PDT (photodynamic therapy)
  - Laser / ablation (also used for tumor in-growth or overgrowth)
  - Radiofrequency ablation
    - APC (argon plasma coagulation)
    - Nd: YAG (neodymium : yttrium-aluminium-garnet)
    - KTP (potassium titanyl phosphate)
- Palliation
  - Ablation (as above)
  - SEMS (self-expanding metal stents (covered for esophagorespiratory fistula)

➢ Radiotherapy
- External beam
  - 3D-CRT (3-dimensional conformal radiotherapy)
  - IMRT (intensity modulated radiotherapy)
- Brachy therapy (with or without concurrent chemotherapy)

➢ Chemoradiotherapy
- Primary (by itself, no surgery)
- With before surgery (neoadjuvant)
  - Concomitant
  - Sequential
- Neoadjuvant chemoradiatherapy with surgery versus surgery alone: RR, all cause, mortality in adeno' or squam' ECa, 0.81

➢ Chemotherapy (metastatic disease)
- Combination therapy:
  - Cisplatinum plus 5-fluorouracil (5-FU) plus epirubicin, or docitaxel
- Biological agents (monoclonal antibody)
  - Cetuximab (anti-EGF receptor)
  - Erlotinib (nati tyrosine kinase)
  - Bevacizumab (anti VEGF)

- Nutrition
    - PEG, percutaneous endoscopic gastrostomy
    - PEJ, percutaneous endoscopic jejunostomy
    - NJ, naso-jejunal tube
    - Parenteral nutrition

- Pain control

- Team care, including palliative care

Abbreviations: EGF, epidermal growth factor; VEGF, vascular endothelial growth factor

Q2. If EUS is superior to CT for staging ECa as well as restaging nodal status of ECa after neoadjuvant preoperative chemoradiotherapy, give the role of FDG PET / CT in restaging ECa.

A2. FDG PET CT is equivalent to EUS and superior to CT alone in evaluating post-chemoradiotherapy status of nodal ECa.

Useful background

Q-point values (overall joint sensitivity-specificity values

FDG PET, 85%
EUS, 86%
CT, 54%

Q3. In the context of esophageal dysphagia, what is the Howel-Evans syndrome?

A3.
- Tylosis, or Howel-Evans syndrome
    - Autosomal dominant
    - GI associations
        - Oral leukoplakia
        - Squamous cell cancer of esophagus (SCCE)
    - Surveillance EGD (for SCCE) age 30, then q 2 years

## Stomach

### 1. Dyspepsia

Q1. In the context of the patient with dyspepsia, diarrhea and flushing, what is the *Darier sign*?

A1. Darier sign is the scratching of the skin causing visible urticaria, resulting from histamine release from mast cells in systemic mastocytosis.

Q2. Dyspepsia associated from hyperchlorhydria is usually treated most efficaciously with PPIs (proton pump inhibitors).

Name the *hypersecretory condition* which responds as well to H2 receptor antagonists as to PPIs, and give the mechanism.

A2. The hyperchlorhydria associated from systemic matocytosis is due to the release of ↑ amounts of histamine from the mast cells. The histamine acts directly on the H2-receptor on the parietal cells, so blocking the H2-receptor with a H2-receptor antagonist is as effective as blocking the proton pumps, because the parietal cells would not be overstimulated by the Achor gastrin receptors.

Q3. On the basis of the G cell, D cell and parietal cells, give the distinction between an H. pyroli infection of the gastric body (*corpus predominant*) versus the gastiic antrum (*antral predominant*)

A3.

- Body predominant gastritis → gastric atrophy → ↓ $H^+$ → ↑ serum gastrin → ↑ PCM (parietal cell mass)

  Antrum predominant gastritis - ↓ D cells → ↓ somatostatin - ↓ inhibition of gastrin release from G cell → ↑ serum gastrin → ↑ HCl

Q4. Give the theoretical basis reflex hyperchlorhydria follwing withdrawal of ↓longterm PPI therapy.

A4.
- PPI → ↓ HCl secretion - ↑ serum gastrin – EC cells hyperplasia and ↑ PCM (hypertrophy)
- When PPI stopped, PCM is hypertrophic, and more HCl may be secreted by unit stimulus

## 2. Gastric air bubble

Q1. What are the cause of an absent *gastric air bubble*?

A1.
- Large hiatus hernia
- Achalasia
- Stomach full of food/fluid
- Large, upper abdominal mass
- Splenomegaly

## 3. Zollinger-Ellison Syndrome

Understanding the physiology of gastrin: a trick – "start with the pathology"

- ZES
  - Uncontrolled ↑ gastrin from gastrinoma
  - ↑ serum gastrin (usually > 1000)
  - ↑ HCl
  - Failure of ↑ HCl to inhibit further release of gastrin (and therefore of HCl) (loss of normal autoregulation)

Positive secretin stimulation test – serum gastrin increases by at least 200 U in response to IV infusion of a weight determined dose of secretin

Q1 In the context of hypergastrinemia, hyperchlorhydria, parietal cell hypertrophy and a positive secretin stimulation test, define the "*gastrinoma triangle*".

A1. The gastrinoma triangle is the anatomical area in which most gastrinomas occur

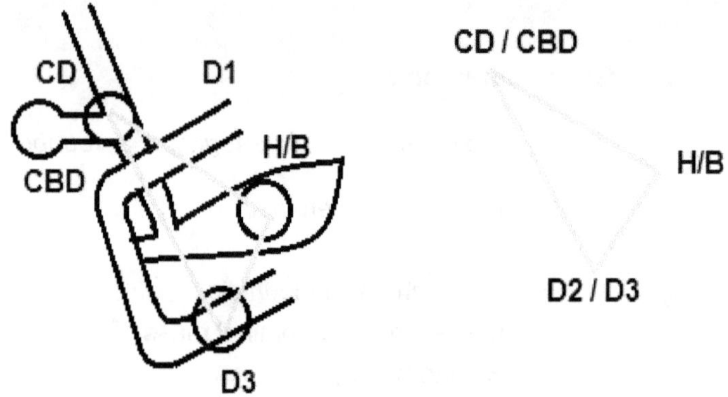


Abbreviation:

- Junction between CD (cystic duct) / CBD (common bile duct)
- Junction between D2 / D3 ($2^{nd}$ and $3^{rd}$ portions of duodenum)
- Junction between H (head) / B (body) of pancreas

Q2. There are numerous clinical features which suggest the Zollinger-Ellison Syndrome (ZES) (Source: Feldman M, et al. *Saunders/Elsevier* 2010, Table 32-6, page 502). About 99% of ZES patients have fasting hypergastrinemia.

Name 2 circumstances where the *fasting gastrin* concentration may be *normal in ZES*.

A2. ○ MEN-1 with hypercalcemia due to

hyperparathyroidism
- Hyperparathyroidectomy may normalize the previously elevated gastrin concentration

- Resection of a gastrinoma may allow the fasting gastrin concentration to normalize (there may still be the possibility that the tumor was not completely resected, and the hypersecretory syndrome may recur).

Q3. In MEN-1-ZES associated hyperparathyroidism, what is the effect of *parathyroidectomy* on gastric physiology?

A3. Parathyroidectomy for hyperthyroidism in MEN-1-ZES has the following benefits:
- ↓ serum calcium
- ↓ fasting gastrin
- ↓ gastrin increase often secretin infusion
- ↓ basal acid output
- ↓ resistance of response to PPIs

Q4. The diagnosis of Zollinger-Ellison Syndrome requires the demonstration of gastric acid hypersecretion in the presence of hypergastrinemia. In ZES, 99% have a gastric pH < 2.

What is the *sensitivity of the measurement of BAO* (basal acid output, mEq/hr) and the secretin provocative test to make the diagnosis of ZES?

A4.
- BAO (mEq/hr)

| | | | | |
|---|---|---|---|---|
| - No previous gastric surgery | >15 | 94%<br>>10 | 90%<br>>15 | 86%<br>>18 |
| - Previous gastric surgery | >5 | 100%<br>>5 | | 73%<br>>14.4 |

- Secretin provocative test
  - Secretin infusion normally ↓ serum gastrin
  - When secretin infusion increases serum gastrin by ≥ 120 pg/ml, the test is positive/ a ZES (sensitivity, 94%; specificity, 100%)

Q5. ZES may be sporatic (S-ZES; 75%), or associated with MEN-1 (*MEN-1-ZES*; 25%). What clinical features suggest MEN-1-ZES rather than *S-ZES*?

A5.
- Renal stones or colic (47% vs 4%)
- Younger age at presentation (34 years vs 43 years)
- Family or personal history of pituitary adenoma or hyperparathyroidism
- 70x greater risk of gastric carcinoids

Q6. We are taught that treatment with proton pump inhibitors do not *cause gastric carcinoid tumors*, but what does the literature on the longterm follow-up of MEN-1-ZES patients treated with PPIs teach us?

A6. In MEN-1-ZES treated with longterm PPIs, half had ECL changes and 23% had gastric carcinoids.

Q7. Gastrin stimulates the growth of the colonic mucosa. What is the prevalence of colorectal carcinoma (*CRC*) in persons with ZES?

A7. Epimoilogic studies have not shown an increased risk of CRC in ZES.

"A straight path never leads anywhere except to the objective"

Andre Gide

## 4. Upper Gastrointestinal bleeding (UGIB)

Q1. What factors would you take into account when *calculating the sample size* for a study of UGIB?

A1.
- MCID (minimal clinically important difference)
- Power
- ARR (absolute risk reduction)
- P value desired
- Size of SD (standard deviation)
- 1- /2- sided
- Surrogate prevalence of outcome validity
- Value of Kappa (inter observer variability (from -1 to +1)

Q2. Give 3 examples of lesions causing UGIB in which *EHT* is not used.

A2. EHT plays no role in the management of UGIB from portal hypertensive gastropathy (ectatic blood vessel), hemobilia, hemosuccus pancreaticus (rupture of splenic artery aneurysm into the pancreatic duct), or aortoenteric fistula.

Q3. Give the three *patterns* of portal hypertensive gastropathy (PHG) seen on EGD.

A3.
- On EGD, PHG appears as
  - Diffuse, subepithelial bleeding giving a red, mosaic pattern to the mucosa (snakeskin appearance)
  - Fine red speckles on the mucosa
  - Red tips of the gastric rugae
- On biopsy of PHG, there are
  - Irregular, tortuous, dilated veins in the mucosa and submucosa
  - Intima thickened
  - No inflammation (no gastritis)

Q4. Give 4 examples of *effective EHT*.

A4.
- o MPEC (multipolar electrocoagulation) probe
- o Injection
- o Hemoclips
- o Band ligation
- o Hemostatic spray
- o Doppler probe ultrasound (cost-minimizing strategy)

Q5. What is the evidence for the use of pre-endoscopy and *pre-EHT PPIs* (proton pump inhibitors)?

A5.
- o Theoretical
- o Cost-effective modeling studies
- o Hong Kong clinical study showing reduction in stigmata of recent bleeding (lower Forrest classification of bleeding source is associated with improved prognosis, i.e. Rebleeding, need for surgery, and mortality)

Q6. Suggest clinical endpoints when *second-look EGD* is indicated for rebleeding after EHT.

A6. Individualize such second-look EGD practice based on the unproven endpoints of

- Clinically apparent recurrent bleeding
- Unexplained low level of hemoglobin concentration after appropriate transfusion
- Hemodynamic instability
- Multiple patient morbidities
- High risk bleeding lesion seen at the index of EGD

Q7. Give 3 methods to *diagnose splenic vein thrombosis* (SVT), which may lead to UGIB from gastric varices.

A7.
- Doppler ultrasound
- MRI
- Angiography

Q8. A cirrhotic patient wishes to be informed about the efficacy of EBL for his bleeding esophageal varices and why he/she is not being offered *sclerotherapy*.

A8.
- Initial homeostasis from EBL of esophageal varices is about 80%, with a rebleeding rate of ~25%.
- EBL is superior to injection therapy in terms of lower rates of rebleeding, overall mortality, as well as mortality from bleeding.
- Just in case he/she asks, efficacy of octreotide for bleeding esophageal varices is similar to balloon tamponade (Sengstaken-Blakemore tube, Minnesota tube, or Linton-Nicholas tube): 90% initial control of bleeding,
- But there are 2 main problems with balloon tamponade
  - > 30% risk of rebleeding once balloon is deflated
  - 30% risk of serious complications

Q9. Compare the efficacy of banding, gluing or injecting *gastric varices from SVT*.

A9. None of these choices is effective!
- The definitive treatment for bleeding gastric varices from SVT is splenectomy.

Q10. If the INR remains prolonged despite administration of FFP (*fresh frozen plasma*) in the cirrhotic patient who is bleeding from esophageal varices, what is the management?

A10. EHT (e.g. EBL) plus 80 µg/kg infusion of human recombinant factor VIIa, plus IV ciprofloxacin 400 mg bid.

Q11. Bad examsmanship – never offer information which you cannot explain an obvious follow-up questions. You said it, so explain the differences between the 3 main types of *balloon tamponade tubes* used for bleeding esophageal varices! (please see above Q/A)

A11.

| | | S-B | MINN | L-N |
|---|---|---|---|---|
| ➢ Balloon | o Esophagus | + | + | - |
| | o Stomach | + | + | + |
| ➢ Aspiration port | o Esophagus | - | + | + |
| | o Stomach | + | + | + |

Abbreviations: L-N, Linton-Nicholas tube; S-B, MINN, Minnesota tube; Sengstaken-Blakemore tube

Q12. Which form of *endoscopic hemostatic therapy* (EHT) provides the more superficial lesion?

A12.
- o Bipolar superficial lesion
- o Hot biopsy, snare deep lesion

Q13. Which form of EHT is best to treat a *re-bleeding ulcer*?

A13. o A clip is preferable to a heater probe.

Q14. Define "Meckel Diverticulum" and give the "rule of two's".

A14. Definition: "Congenital blind intestinal pouch that results from incomplete obliteration of the vitelline duct during gestation".

Source: Feldman M, et al. *Saunders/Elsevier* 2010, page 317.

- Rules of 2's
  - Prevalence
  - Distance from ileocecal valve
  - Length, inches
  - Complications
  - Types of ectopic mucosa (gastric, pancreatic)
  - Age by which child usually presents age
  - Ratio of males to females

Source: Feldman M, et al. *Saunders/Elsevier* 2010, page 318.

Q15. Give the clinical, etiological, pathological and complication differences in HHT (hereditary hemorrhagic telangiectasia, aka *Osler-Weber-Rendu disease*), and angiectasias (AEs).

A15.
- ➢ The lesions of HHT do involve the lips, mouth, nose, fingers. The Curacao criteria need to be fulfilled to make a clinical diagnosis of HHT.
  - Telangiectasias
  - Epistaxis
  - Visceral lesions
  - Family history

- Etiology
    - Molecular genetic studies demontrate an autosomal dominant disorder in which there are two possible mutations of the HHT genes (genetypic heterogeneity).
        - ENG gene mutations
        - Encodes for endoglin, a TGF-β receptor
        - Type 2 : Activin receptor-like kinase-1 gene mutation
        - Encodes for ACVRL, protein, also a TGF-β receptor

- Pathology
    - Site
        - Stomach
        - Small bowel
        - Colon (AEs mostly in colon and small bowel)
    - Irregular, dilated, tortuous spaces
    - Single layer of endothelial cells
    - Vessels lack elastic lamina or muscular lissue
    - Arterioles
        - Thrombi (vascular stasis)
        - Proliferation of the intima
    - Venules
        - Thick wall (recall that the wall of venules in AE is thin)

- Complications
    - Involvement of lungs, brain and spinal cord, liver
    - High flow in vessels may lead to
        - High output congestive heart failure
        - Portal hypertension and liver failure

## 5. Bariatric surgery

Q1. Give reasons why an EGD is recommended for all persons prior to bariatric surgery.

A1.

- High risk of treatable lon

| | % | | % |
|---|---|---|---|
| - Esophagus | | | |
| GERD | | | |
| ▪ LA A to D | 3.7 | ▪ Gastric carcinoid | 0.3 |
| ▪ BE | 3.7 | ▪ Multiple lesions | 1.1 |
| - Stomach/ duodenum | | | |
| ▪ Erosive gastritis | 1.8 | | |
| ▪ GU | 2.9 | | |
| ▪ DU | 0.7 | | |

- High risk of a symptomatic lesions - 1/3 of bariatric patients had a symptomatic pre-operative lesions
- Difficult post-surgical investigation of upper GI tract with RNYGB

Abbreviation: BE, barrett epithelium; DU, duodenal ulcer; EGD, esophagogastroduodenoscopy; GERD, gastroesophageal reflux disease; GU, gastric ulcer; RNYGB, Roux-on-Y gastric bypass

Q2. *Draw* the four most commonly performed *gastric bypass procedures.*

A2.

- Malabsorptive
  - BPD-DS (biliopancreatic diversion-duodenal switch)
- Restrictive
  - LABG (laparoscopic adjustable banding gastroplasty)
  - VBG (vertical banded gastroplasty)
- Restrictive and malabsorptive
  - RNYGB (Roux-en-Y gastric bypass

For more details, see: Feldman M, et al. *Saunders/Elsevier* 2010, Figure 7.1, page 116.

Q3. It is widely accepted that there is proven efficacy of bariatric surgery (RNYGB, VBG, LAGB and BPD-DS) in the areas of excess weight loss (EWL), mortality and resolution of comorbidities.

Give the *approximate rates of improvement*, in the mortality rates, of obesity-associated co-morbidities.

A3.

- % ↓ mortality from RNYGB
  - Coronary artery disease 56
  - Diabetes 92
  - Cancer, all types 60
  - Obesity – associated cancers
    - Esophagus 2
    - Colon 30
    - Breast 9
    - Uterus 78
    - NHL 46
    - MM 54

- % resolution of *comorbidities* (approximate)

| | Hypertension | Diabetes | Hyperlipidemia |
|---|---|---|---|
| RNYGB | 70 | 82 | 63 |
| BPD-DS | 81 | 98 | 99 |
| Banding | 38 | 48 | 71 |
| Gastroplasty | 73 | 68 | 81 |
| Bypass | 75 | 84 | 94 |

- Additional improvements
  - Q of L (SF 36 survey)
  - Resolution of GERD symptoms (may occur postoperatively)
  - NASH, % histological improvements
    - Steatosis 90
    - Hepatocellular ballooning 59
    - Centrilobular-perisinusoidal fibrosis 50

Source: Feldman M, et al. *Saunders/Elsevier* 2010, page 116-118

Q4. Give the *NIH consensus criteria* for persons to qualify for bariatric surgery:

A4.
- Without obesity – related co – morbidities: BMI > 40 kg/m$^2$
- With obesity – related co – morbidities: BMI > 35 40 kg/m$^2$
- Pre-operative weight loss is not part of the NIH criteria, but this is associated with shorter operative times, and greater weight loss at one year after surgery

## 6. Abdominal pain and masses

Q1. A sexually active woman of reproductive potential presents with acute abdominal pain three weeks after a *missed menses*. What are the most likely diagnoses?

A1.
- Ectopic pregnancy
- PID (pelvic inflammatory disease)
- Ovarian cyst or tortion

Adapted from: Filate W, et al. *The Medical Society, Faculty of Medicine, University of Toronto* 2005, page 37.

Q2. How can you attempt to differentiate between *involuntary or malingering pain*?

A2. Try to distract patient by pretending to auscultate but pushing in the stethoscope, and watch the patient's face for signs of discomfort

Q3. *Hyperalgesia and allodynia* are both types of pain, but differ in the type of signal bringing on the pain; give the signal which causes the pain in each of these.

A3.

| Word | ↑ pain response to signal |
|---|---|
| o Hyperalgesia | - Noxious |
| o Allodynia | - Non-noxious |

Q4. Which portions of the visceral pain transmission to the CNS are abnormal / dysfunctional in IBS?

A4.
- ACC (anterior cingulate cortex)
- PACC (perigenual ACC)
- Dorsal ACC
- MCC (mid cingulate cortex)

Q5. Give the main mediators of the *stress-immune response.*

A5.
- CRF (corticotropin releasing factor)
- HPA (hypothalamic-pituitary-adrenal axis)
- Pro-inflammatory cytokines
- Locus-coeruleus-norepinephrine) systems in CNS

## 7. Appendicitis and peritonitis

Q1. In the context of abdominal pain and tenderness, what are the *Hover, Carnett and Jump signs*?

A1.
- Hover – the patient "hovers" their hand (s) over the abdomen during physical examination of the abdomen
- Carnet - ↑ tenderness of the abdominal call to palpation when the patient voluntarily tenses the muscles of the abdominal wall
- Jump – A negative reaction ("jump") made by the patient when the abdominal wall is examined
  - The trigger point may be only the size of a finger tip

Q2. In the context of the patient with intra-abdominal pathology, what is the Kehr sign, and what is its mechanism?

A2.
- With any cause of irritation of the diaphragm, for example from a subdiaphragmatic abscess or hematoma, or splenic rupture, the pain may be referred to the left shoulder.
- "Referred pain is ordinarily located in the cutaneous dermatomes that share the same spinal cord level as the affected visceral inputs" (Yarze JC & Friedman LS. Sleisenger and Fordtran's Gastrointestinal and Liver Disease. 9th Edition. *Saunders/Elsevier* 2010, page 163)
- First – order visceral afferent neuron from splenic rupture synapses
- With both first – order somatic afferent neuron as well as second – order spinal cord neuron.

## 8. Intra-abdominal abscess (IAA)

Q1. Give 10 bacterial adjuvant or host defense factors influencing the *transition* from bacterial contamination to infection.

A1.

- Bacterial Factors
  - Adherence capacity
  - Invasiveness
  - Metabolic systems
  - Resistance to antibiotics
- Adjuvant Factors
  - Barium
  - Blood
  - Fecal matter
  - Fibrin
  - Foreign material
  - Necrotic tissue
- Host Defense Factors
  - Fibrin sequestration
  - Lymphatic clearance
  - Neutrophil influx
  - Lymphocyte response
  - Peritoneal macrophages

Printed with permission: Feldman M, et al. *Saunders/Elsevier* 2010, Table 26-3, page 412.

Q2. Give 5 causes of intra-abdominal abscesses (IAA), and 7 *clinical risk factors.*

A2.

- Causes of IAA
  - Stomach/ abdomen
    - Penetration / perforation
  - Small bowel
    - Crohn disease
  - Colon
    - Crohn disease
    - Diverticulitis

- Neoplastic disease
- Appendix
  - Appendicitis
- Gallbladder
  - Cholecystectomy operations
- Pancreas
  - Pancreatitis
- General
  - Abdominal trauma
  - Perforated hollow viscous (e.g., duodenal or gastric ulcer)

Source: Feldman M, et al. *Saunders/Elsevier* 2010, Table 26-1, page 412.

- Clinical Risk Factors for IAA
  - Systemic Factors
    - Chronic glucocorticoid use
    - Increasing age
    - Malnutrition
    - Preexisting organ dysfunction
    - Transfusion
    - Malignancy
  - Local Factors
    - Delay in performing surgery for underlying disease
    - Formation of an ostomy
    - Nonappendiceal source of infection
    - Severe of illness, infection
    - Severe of trauma

Source: Feldman M, et al. *Saunders/Elsevier* 2010, Table 26-2, page 412.

Q3. Give the *abdominal diagnostic imaging* findings suggestive of the presence of IAA.

A3.
- Plain films
  - Mass effect
  - Extraluminal gas
  - Localized ileus

- Ultrasound
  - Round/oval mass with
    - ↓central echogenicity (fluid, gas)
    - Thick wall
    - Internal debris

*Note: false negative findings may be due to overlying bowel gas blocking ultrasound waves

- Computed tomography (*CT) scan*
  - Extraluminal mass homogeneous fluid density, or heterogeneous solid density if IAA contains phlegmon
  - Extraluminal gas
  - Thick wall enhancement
  - Adjacent inflammatory changes

- Gallium 67 ($^{67}$Ga) or nuclear imaging scanning
  - Useful to follow-up CT scan

- Magnetic resonance imaging (MRI)
  - Limited use

## 9. Abdominal aorta

Q1. About 3 persons in 4 have the classic triad for ruptures of a "*triple A"* (AAA, abdominal aortic aneurysm). Give the components of this triad:

A1.
- Abdominal pain
- Tender, pulsatile abdominal mass
- Hypotension

Q2. What are the names of the two signs of abdominal wall discolouration which suggest the presence of an *ectopic pregnancy* and *ruptured AAA*?

A2.
- Cullen Sign: Purple-blue discoloration around umbilicus peritoneal hemorrhage; caused by acute pancreatitis or ectopic pregnancy (cullen sign occurs in the centre of the abdomen)

- Grey-Turner Sign: Flank discolouration retroperitoneal hemorrhage Grey-Turner sign is in the flanks and is best seen when you turn the patient; caused by
  - acute pancreatitis
  - ruptured abdominal aortic aneurysm (AAA)
  - strangulated bowel

Adapted from: Filate W, et al. *The Medical Society, Faculty of Medicine, University of Toronto* 2005, page 37.

## 10. Tumors and Polyps

Q1. Give the types of inherited familial neuroendocrine tumors (*F-NETs*), for which family screening may be appropriate.

A1.
- MEN-1 (Werner syndrome)
- Tuberous sclerosis
- Neurofibromatosis-1 (Von Hippel-Lindau disease)

Q2. In the 25% of gastric MALT which show *non - response to H. pylori eradication*, what are the explanations?

A2. May be due to

- One of the chromosomal translocations [t (11, 18)], as suggested by IHC staining for nuclear BCL-10.
- Possibly due to expression of Cag A protein.
- High grade and/or extensive disease.

- Gastric H. Pylori infection causes chronic gastritis, an immune response which attracts T and B cells to the gastric mucosa. The T cells and the B cells proliferate during this T cell-dependent B-cell response to the H. Pylori.
- B cell monoclonality develops.
- These lymphomas cells invade the lamina propria, grow around reactive follicles, and invade the germinal centres (follicular colonization); MALT lymphoma results.

Q3. Half of gastric lymphomas are MALT with diffused superficial gastric infiltration, and the remainder are DLBCL (diffuse large B cell tumor masses, with areas of marginal zone-MALT-type lymphoma).

What is the use of PET scans to distinguish between the diffuse superficial gastric infiltration of MALT lymphoma, versus the masses seen in diffuse large B cell (*DLBCL*) lymphoma?

A3. Very little of fluorodeoxyglucose ($^{18}$F-FDG) used for PET scanning is taken up by gastric lymphomas, so better do EGD plus biopsy, EUS or CT scan.

- Incontrast to the > 90% association of MALT lymphoma with H. pylori, with DLBCL the association is only absent one third, even if MALT and DLBCL co-exist.

Q4. Give the histology of *PETs*.

A4.
- Sheets of homogeneous, small round cells
- Uniform nuclei and cytoplasm
- High vascularity
- Few mitotoc figures

Q5. Give the differences on *EUS* of benign versus malignant GIST in mid-stomach.

A5.

| Characteristics | Benign | Malignant |
|---|---|---|
| ➢ Echo texture | Homogeneous | Heterogeneous |
| ➢ Margins | Regular | Irregular |
| ➢ Cystic spaces | - | + |
| ➢ Size | < 3 cm | > 4 cm |
| ➢ Associated lymph node | - | + |

Q6. A patient with chronic dyspepsia on PPI therapy has a family history of colonic polyps. Your patient has a normal colonoscopy, but shows multiple *fundic gland polyps* (FGP). Biopsy of these polyps shows
- Cystic dilations of oxyntic gland mucosa
- Reduced numbers of parietal, chief and mucous neck cells

Give the *immunological staining* that should be performed to distinguished sporatic from familial FGPs.

A6. ➢ Sporatic
- Mutations of B-catenin gene
- Enhanced growth with PPIs
- May be associated with APC gene alterations when there is associated dysplasia (3%)

- Familial
  - Usually have APC gene alterations on chromosome 5
  - Colonic polyps do not necessarily develop (i.e. characteristic FAP)
  - Dysplasia in 25%

Q7. Give the mechanism for the development of hypernatremia, hypokalemia, hypochloremic, metabolic alkalosis (↑ $Na^+$, ↓ $K^+$, ↑ $Cl^-$, ↑ $HCO_3^-$) which occur with *gastric outlet obstruction*.

A7.
- Gastric outlet obstruction → vomiting HCl
- $HCO_3^-$ secreted by pancreas and by parietal cell basolateral membrane ("alkaline tide")
- The $HCO_3^-$ is not nebulized by HCl, since HCl was lost by vomiting.
- The resulting metabolic causes $H^+$ reabsorption and $K^+$ loss by the renal NHE ($Na^+$ / $H^+$ exchanger).
- Vomiting causes dehydration, which leads to $Na^+$ and more $K^+$ loss through the $Na^+$ / $K^+$ exchanger
- Dehydration causes ↑BUN

Q8. Name 4 cell types of *endocrine tumors* of the stomach.

A8.
- ECL (histamine-producing enterochromaffin-like) cells in the gastric body and fundus
- G (gastrin producing) cells in the antrum
- D (somatostatin-producing) cells (a subset may contain calcitonin, PP and ACTH
- P (ghrelin-producing) cells
- EC (serotonin-producing enterochromaffin) cells

## 11. Diagnostic Imaging

Give the Distinguishing diagnoses on Diagnostic Imaging

- Gastric mass with central ulceration
  - Adenocarcinoma
  - Lymphoma
  - GIST
  - Metastatic melanoma
  - Ectopic pancreatic rest

- Central depression / ulceration
  - Malignant GIST
  - Lipoma
  - Ectopic pancreatic rest (umbilication; not an ulcer, since surface is covered with normal epithelium)
  - Metastatic melanoma

- Lymphoma versus adenocarcinoma

| | Lymphoma | Adenocarcinoma |
|---|---|---|
| Number | Single or multiple | Single |
| Extent | Extensive | Localized |
| Origin | Submucosa | Mucosa |
| Cross pylorus | Yes | No |
| Narrowed lumen | No | Yes |
| Distensible | Yes | No |
| Disorganized | Yes | - |

## Small bowel

### 1. Intraluminal duodenal diverticula

Q1. In the context of duodenal diverticula, what is "*windsox diverticula*".

A1.
- Windsox or intraluminal duodenal diverticula are single sac-like structures that arise from $D_2$ (the second portion of the diverticulum), and are attached to part or the entire circumference of the duodenal wall.
- Both sides of the diverticular are lined by mucosa
- If a diverticulum is inverted in an erect direction and is viewed by EGD, it will appear as a mass.

### 2. Crohn Disease

Q1. Give 6 prognostic indicators of successful *spontaneous fistula closure*.

A1.

| Parameter | Spontaneous Closure Likely |
|---|---|
| ➢ Nutritional status | o Well nourished |
| ➢ Cause | o Anastomotic breakdown |
| | o No malignancy, inflammatory or infectious disease, or complete anastomotic dehiscence |
| ➢ Anatomic characteristics | o Long fistulous tract |
| | o No eversion of mucosa |
| ➢ Duration | o Acute |

| Parameter | Spontaneous Closure Likely |
|---|---|
| ➢ Output (mL/day) | ○ <500 |
| ➢ Age (yr) | ○ <40 |
| ➢ Site | ○ Proximal small bowel |

### 3. Infection

Q1. In the patient with unexplained chronic diarrhea, you resort to the measurement of the osmotic gap determined on a spot collection of stool. Show how to calculate the *stool osmotic gap* (SOG). In the patient with SOG > 50 mOSm/kg, you return to the history: give substances which can cause chronic diarrhea when SOG > 50.

A1.
- ➢ Stool osmotic gap (SOG) = 290 – 2 ($Na_s^+$ + $K_s^+$)
  $Na_s^+$, stool $Na_s^+$; $K_s^+$, stool $K^+$
  - ○ Abnormal SOG ≥ 50 mOsm/kg
- ➢ Commonly ingested substances causing chronic (osmotic) diarrhea with SOG > 50

| | |
|---|---|
| ○ Carbohydrates | - Lactose – milk<br>- Sucrose-pop, sweeteners<br>- Fructose |
| ○ Magnesium-laxatives | - Sorbitol – chewing gum, diabetic candy<br>- Lactulose – laxative<br>- Trehalose - mushrooms |

## 4. Lymphoma

Q1. A small bowel barium study reports a curious bull's eye lesion. MR enteroscopy demonstrates a small bowel tumor. The diagnostic imager suggests the lesion may be a metastasis.
Give the primary cancers which spead directly, by seeding or by lymphatic spread to the GI tract.

A1.

| Metastatic Site | Primary |
|---|---|
| ➢ Esophagus | ○ Stomach<br>○ Lung |
| ➢ Stomach | ○ Breast |
| ➢ Pancreas | ○ Lung<br>○ Kidney<br>○ Luminal GI |
| ➢ Small bowel | ○ Stomach<br>○ Pancreas<br>○ Biliary tree<br>○ Kidney<br>○ Retroperitoneum<br>○ Melanoma |

## 5. Gastrointestinal stroma tumors (GIST)

Q1. What IHC stains help to distinguish GISTs, leiomyosarcomas and schwannomas?

A1.
- Leiomyosarcomas-positive for both SMA (smooth muscle actin) and desmin, negative for CD117
- Schwannomas-positive for S100 (a neural antigen), CD117 negative
- Recall that GISTs are usually (>95%) CD117 positive

Q2. About 5% of GISTs are KIT-negative. What is the *non-KIT signal* for these GISTs?

A2. Mutational activation and aberrant signaling from PDGFRA (platelet-derived growth factor receptor-alpha)

Q3. What are the three most common NETs (carcinoid tumors) in the duodenum?

A3.

- Gastrin, 70%
- Somatostatin, 25%
- Gangliocytic paraganglioma, 5% (a benign humartoma)

Q4. Give 3 *cytosolic markers* for poorly differentiated GI-NET.

A4.

- NSE
- PEP 9.5
- Synaptophysin (marker for synaptic-like vesicles)

Q5. There are 3 types of gastric carcinoid tumors (NET), type I, II, and III. For type I and II, there is a slow rate of metastasis to the liver and lymph nodes, so the survival rate is very good; the cell of the origin is ECL (rather than EC for the type III); there may be more than one tumor; the tumors are usually < 1 cm in size and there is hypergastrinemia.

Give 3 pathological features which help to distinguish the type III sporatic tumors from the type I and II gastric NETs.

A5.

| Associated gastric pathology | I AMAG | II HG | III N/NS |
|---|---|---|---|
| o Antral G-cell hyperplasia | + | - | - |
| o ECL hyperplasia | + | + | - |

Abbreviations: AMAG, autoimmune metaplastic atrophic gastritis; HG, hypertrophic gastropathy; N/NS, normal or non-specific changes

Source: Feldman M, et al. *Saunders/Elsevier* 2010, Table 31-2, page 479.

Q6. GI NETs are associated with gene point mutations, deletions, methylation, as well as chromosomal gains and losses.

Give 3 examples of the *genetic changes* in GI-NET

A6.

- Fore-gut (stomach)
  - MENIN gene (tumor suppressor gene), common in MEN-1 syndrome
  - MENIN intracts with numerous factors such as the AP1 transcription factor, JUN D and NF-κβ
  - Loss of heterozygosity on chromosome II in MEN-1 gene
- Mid-gut (small intestine)
  - Deletions on chromosome 18
- Hind-gut (colon)
  - TGF-α
  - EGF
- Others
  - NAPILI
  - MAGE D2
  - MTA1

## 6. Diarrhea and Malabsorption

Q1. Give 3 factors associated with the ↑ risk of *pneumatosis intestinalis* in SOT (solid organ transplant).

A1.
- Infection
  - CMV
  - C. difficile
- Drug / toxins
  - Steroids

Q2. EBV does not usually form mucosal ulcers and cause GI tract bleeding. What is the exception to this "*rule*"?

A2. When EBV-LPD (lymphoproliferative disease) develops, ulceration and bleeding may occur. This is the cause of PTLD (post-transplant lymphoprolifertive disorder, a B or T cell lymphoma, and may require reduction of immunosuppression, rituximab.

Q3. *Medullary carcinoma* of the thyroid (MCT) is often associated with diarhea. Give 4 causes of diarrhea in MCT which are related to this condition.

A3.
- ↑ calcitonin
- ↑ VIP
- ↑ prostaglandins
- ↑ rate of colonic transit (etiology not yet known)
- Men II
  - A. hyperparathyroidism (usually causes constipation, rather than diarrhea)
  - Pheochromocytomas

Q4. Apolipoprotein B is contained in chylomicrons, LDL (low density lipoprotein) and VLDL (very low density lipoproteins). Lack of apoprotein B results in a recessive disorder, *abetalipoproteinemia*. Abetalipiproteinemia is characterized by steatorrhea, ataxia, atypical acanthosis pigmentosa, acanthotic red blood cells, and absence in the serum of chylomicrons, LDL and VLDL.

Give the *histological features* of abetalipoproteinemia seen on small bowel biopsy.

A4.

- Mucosal cells
  - Abundant lipid droplets
- Submucosa and lamina propria
  - Little lipid
- Lipoprotein
  - Empty

Q5 The 1 year risk of *recurrence of C. difficile* is 25%. If the patient has experienced one relapse, what is the risk of a further relapse?

A5. After a previous relapse, the risk of a future relapse is 50%.

Q6. What is the *risk of giving probiotics* to a patient with a severe C.diff. infection?

A6. Probiotics may cause bacteremia when given to the patient with severe C.diff. infection.

## 7. Umbilicus

Q1. What are the uses of examining the "*belly button*"?

A1.
- Direction of flow of blood in veins of abdominal wall-flow below umbilicus is down into saphenous veins, above umbilicus is upwards into veins of thoracic wall. In portal hypertension, dilated veins show normal direction of flow, but in IVC obstruction, flow in veins below umbilicus is reversed, i.e. Flows upward.
- Umbilicus is common site of infiltration by cancer metastases (Sister Mary Joseph's nodule)
- Protuberance from ascites (an "out-ie")

## 8. Celiac disease

Q1. What qualifies as a "*gluten-free diet*"?

A1. A diet with < 20 ppm gluten qualifies as being "gluten free".

## 9. Diagnostic Imaging

Give the Distinguishing diagnoses on Diagnostic Imaging

- Multiple, duodenal filling defects
  - Fundic gland polypopsis syndrome (FAP)
  - Gastric polyps hyperplastic
  - Duodenal polyps adenomatous

- Smooth-surfaced filling defects
  - Inflammatory fibroid polyp
  - GIST
  - Lipoma
  - Hemagioma
- Dilation of proximal small bowel / duodenum
  - Superior mesenteric artery (SMA) syndrome
  - AAA (abdominal aortic aneurysm)
  - Duodenal neoplasia
  - Pancreatitis
- Narrowing
  - Focal infilterative lymphoma
    - Loss of mucosal folds in narrow lumen
  - Ischemia
  - Amyloidosis
    - Secondary ischemic changes (loss of mucosal folds)
    - Thickening of small bowel folds
- Multiple filling defects
  - Lymphoma
  - Hemangioma
  - Neurofibroma
  - Metastases
  - Multiple intestinal polyposis
  - Polyposis syndrome
- Lipoma versus liposarcoma
  - Liposarcoma
    - heterogeneous fat density
    - soft tissue in tumor
- Polypoid mass (any submucosal tumor)
  - Lipoma
  - GIST

- Multiple masses in a single loop of bowel
  - Lymphoma
  - Metastases

- Metastasis to the bowel wall, growing into the mesentery and destroying the bowel wall, leading to loss of mucosa
  - Lymphoma
  - GIST
  - Metastases from colon

- Whipple disease
  - Mycobacterium avium-intracellular (MAC)
  - Giardiasis
  - Cryptosporosis

- Indistinguishable from Crohn disease (erosions, fold thickening, strictures)
  - Tuberculosis
  - Actinomycosis
  - Histoplasmosis
  - Blastomycosis

- Isolated small bowel ulcers
  - Nonspecific (idiopathic)
  - Infection
    - TB
  - Immune
    - Behcet syndrome
    - Celiac disease
  - Ischemia
  - Heterotropic gastric mucosa
  - Trauma
  - Drugs
    - Arsenic

## Colon

### 1. LGIB (Lower GI Bleeding)

Q1. Why are *colonic diverticulae* misnamed?

A1. Colonic diverticulae are ".....herniations of colonic mucosa and submucosa through the muscular layer of colon...at points of entry of the small arteries (Vasa Recta)." (Feldman M, et al. *Saunders/Elsevier* 2010, page 311). Because these "diverticular" do not contain all layers of the colonic wall, they are actually pseudodiverticular.

Q2. Give 4 risk factors for PPB (*post polypectomy bleeding*).

A2.

- polyp
  - > 2 cm
  - Thick stalk
  - Sessile
  - Right colon
- Patient
  - Use of ASA, NSAID, anticoagulant

Source: Feldman M, et al. *Saunders/Elsevier* 2010, page 313.

Q3. Give the blood supply of *rectal varices*.

A3. "Ectopic varices may develop in the rectal mucosa between the superior hemorrhoidal veins (portal circulation) in persons with portal hypertension"

Source: Feldman M, et al. *Saunders/Elsevier* 2010, page 314.

Q4. Define severe LGIB, give the predictors of severe LGIB, and the predictors of in hospital mortality.

A4. ➢ Definition

- Continued bleeding within the first 24 hours of hospitalization
  - Transfusion of ≥ 2 units PRBC, ±
  - ≥ 20% ↓ hematocrit, ±
- Recurrent bleeding after 24 hours of stability
  - Need for additional transfusions
  - ≥ 20% further ↓ hematocrit, or
  - Readmission to hospital for LGIB within 1 week of discharge

Source: Feldman M, et al. *Saunders/Elsevie* 2010, page 309.

Q5. Give 4 disadvantages of *angiography* done for LGIB (lower GI bleeding).

A5.

- Positive results in only ~ half of patients (bleeding may intermittent, or too slow [requires arterial bleeding rate of > 0.5 ml/min])
- Complication rate 3% to 10%
  - Bowel
    - Ischemia
    - Hematoma
  - Femoral artery thrombosis
  - Reactions to contrast dye
    - Acute renal damage
  - TIAs (transient [cerebral] ischemic attacks)
- Multi-detector CT is more accurate than technetium-tagged RBC in LGIB
- Colonoscopy is of limited use in LGIB, visualizing presumed or definite causes in only about 2/3's

Q6. Give 4 angiographic signs of AEs (angioectasias).

A6. The important angiographic signs of AEs include:

- Dilated, tortuous vains, which are slow to empty the angiographic dye
- Vascular tuft
- Early filling vein
- Extravasation of contrast material

Q7. In the context of lower gastrointestinal intestinal bleeding (LGIB), what is *Heyde syndrome*?

A7. Heyde syndrome is LGIB from colonic angiodysplasia in the patient with aortic sclerosis, thought to be due to 'proteolysis of the largest multimers of the Von Willebrand factor' (Feldman M, et al. *Saunders/Elsevier* 2010, page 584)

## 2. Constipation

Q1. Give a clinical classification of the mechanisms of *functional constipation*.

A1.

| | |
|---|---|
| o Normal – transit constipation | |
| o Slow-transit constipation (STC) | - Colonic retention of > 20% of radiopaque markers at day 5 post ingestion |
| o Defecatory disorders | - Abnormal balloon expulsion test, ± <br> - Abnormal rectal manometry |

Q2. Give 4 abnormalities of colonic function in patients with STC (*slow-transit constipation*).

A2.
- ↓ HAPCs (high – amplitude propagated contractions)
- ↓ SP (substance P, an excitatory transmitter)
- ↑ VIP (vasoactive intestinal polypeptide) and NO (nitric oxide) (inhibitory transmitters)
- ↓ number & abnormalities of ICCs (interstitial cells of Cajal)
- ↓ number of myenteric ganglion cells

Q3. From the lateral view of the rectum on barium enema examination, what are the features that suggest the *descending perineum syndrome*?

A3.
- Rectum is more vertical than is normal
- The anorectal angle is wide
- Perineal discent is > 3 cm

Q4. What is thought to be the pathophysiology of the *solitary rectal ulcer syndrome* (SRUS)?

A4. SRUS is thought be caused by paroxysmal contraction of the puborectalis muscle from excessive straining during defecation.

Q5. What is the pathophysiology of constipation occurring in *hypothyroidism*?

A5.
- Myxedematous infiltration in the wall of the colon
- Reduced peristalsis

Q6. The *colon transit time* (CTT) is ~12 hours. What does the measurement of CTT indicate about the pathophysiology of constipation?

A6. CTT is delayed in transit disorders, whereas in defecatory disorders of the rectoanal inhibitory reflex or pelvic floor dysfunction (anismus), there will be a hold-up of fecal marks in the rectal area.

## 3. Laxatives

Q1. Give a *mechanistic classification of laxatives*, and for each give an example.

A1.

- Osmotic
  - Magnesium, sulfate, phosphate
  - Lactulose, sorbitol, mannitol, PEG (polyethylene glycol)
- Stimulant
  - Anthraquinones: senna, cascara
  - Ricinoleic acid: castor oil
  - Diphenylmethanes: phenolphthalein, bisacodyl, sodium picosulfate
- Prokinetics
  - Cisapride, tegaserod
- Softeners
  - Sodium docusate
- Lubricants
  - Mineral oil
- Locally acting
  - Suppositories, glycerin, bisacodyl
  - Enemas tap water, soap suds, phosphate, mineral oil
- Chloride channel activator
  - Lubiprostone

*Note: in extreme circumstances laparoscopic open subtotal colectomy with ileorectal anastomosis may be necessary for severe constipation.

Q2. There are many laxatives which are available to treat chronic constipation. For which of these is their used based on two or more randomized controlled trials (*RCTs*) with adequate sample sizes and appropriate methodology?

A2. Lactulose, PEG, Tegaserod®.

## 4. Diarrhea

Q. Give five clinical and/or laboratory features which increase the pretest probability that a patient's chronic diarrhea is *factitious* and caused by surreptitious laxative abuse.

A.

- Demographic groups
  - Female
  - Health care worker
  - Secondary gain
  - History of
    - Bulimia
    - Munchausen syndrome
    - Polle syndrome (Munchausen syndrome by proxy (dependent child or adult poisoned with laxatives by parent or caregiver)
- Serum
  - Hypokalemia (senna)
- Stool
  - ↑ fecal osmotic gap
  - ↑/ ↓ osmolality (addition of hypertonic urine, or of water)
- Sigmoid mucosa
  - Pseudomelanosis coli (anthracene laxative abuse)

## 5. Ischemia

Q1. When ischemic changes are seen in the wall of the colon, what are the histopathological features which suggest a *microangiopathic antiphospholipid* – associated disorder?

A1.
- o Vasculitis
- o Deposits of immune complexes
- o C3 complement
- o Fibrinogen

Q2. How are your $10^{14}$ cells today?

A2. They are fine, but I am experiencing destructive interference from my $10^{15}$ gut microbiotica cells!

Q3. Funny! We all know what are probiotics, prebiotics and symbiotics. What are *bacteriocins*?

A3. Bacteriocins are substances that are produced by some bacteria which modify the growth of other bacteria.

## 6. Infections

Q1. Give the antibiotic recommended for the treatment of hemorrhagic colitis due to *E. coli O157.H7* infection.

A1. There is none; in fact, antibiotic treatment of E. coli O157.H7 may precipitate HUS-TTS (hemorrhagic uremic syndrome and thrombotic thrombocytopenic purpura).

## 7. Obstruction / Pseudo-obstruction

Q1 Define "*Ogilvie Syndrome*", and give 4 of its commonly associated causative conditions.

A1. Definition: Ogilvie Syndrome is acute colonic pseudo-obstruction. "......characterized by marked dilation of the cecum [> 10 cm] and ascending colon in the absence of mechanical obstruction" (Spiegel, BMR, et al. *Slack Incorporated* 2011, page 110).

- Common associations
    - ICU patients
    - Sepsis
    - Recent surgery
    - Electrolyte abnormalities
    - Trauma
    - Drugs
    - Immobilization

## 8. Diverticulitis

Q1. Outline the treatment of acute diverticulitis, based on the Hinchey grading system of abdominal CT.

A1.

| Hinchey CT grade | | Treatment |
|---|---|---|
| 0 | Perforation and no comorbidity | - Outpatient oral antibiotics |
| I | Abscess pericolic/ pericolic inflammation | - IV antibiotics |
| II | Abscess (pelvis, abdomen, retroperitoneal) | - IV antibiotics<br>- CT – guided drainage of abscess |
| II | Generalized purulent peritonitis | - Surgery |
| IV | Generalized fecal peritonitis | |

## 9. Colorectal cancer (CRC)

Q1. Give reasons why the risk of colorectal cancer is increased two-fold in *acromegaly*.

A1.
- ↑ incidence of colonic adenomatous polyps
- These adenomatous polyps are often
  - Large
  - Multiple
  - Right-sided (possibly more difficult to see on colonoscopy)

## 10. Colitis

Q1. What are the three *histological features* which are used to distinguish chronic from acute colitis?

A1. Chronic colitis has three features which distinguish it from acute colitis:
- Branched crypts
- Inflammatory gap
- Paneth cell metaplasia

## 11. Typhlitis

Q1 If the CT scan shows thickening of the bowel wall of the appendix, terminal ileum or cecum, *typhlitis* may be suspected.

Give the clinical and laboratory abnormalities which should alert you to this diagnostic possibility, and state why this diagnosis must not be missed.

A1.
- Typhlitis is also known as neutropenic enterocolitis with most of the conditions in the differential, the WBC would be increased or at least normal. If the neutrophil count is low, then consider this diagnosis.
- Typhlitis is highly prone to perforate (mortality rate, 50%) because of the necrotizing nature of the process. Because of this, colonoscopy or barium enema studies should be avoided.

## 12. Diagnostic Imaging

Give the Distinguishing diagnoses on Diagnostic Imaging

- Scleroderma colon vs Crohn colitis

| | Scleroderma colon | Crohn colitis |
|---|---|---|
| o Patchy (segmental) | + | + |
| o Mesenteric border | + | - |
| o Antimesenteric border | + | + |

- CT of stool
  - Inhomogeneous
  - Air / fat attenuation
  - Moves
- Lipoma vs. serosal metastasis

| | Lipoma | serosal metastasis |
|---|---|---|
| o Multiple | - | + |
| o Tethering | - | + |

- Multiple filling defects
  - Polyposis syndrome polyps
    - Larger
    - Variable size
    - Pedunculated
  - Crohn colitis aphthous ulcers
    - Distribution
      - Patchy
      - Segmental
  - Diffuse lymphoma
    - Larger ( > 4 mm diameter)
    - Nodules
      - Smooth
      - Round
    - Variable size
  - Retained stool
    - Angular margins
    - Moves

## Liver

### 1. Alcohol Abuse

Q1. In the context of alcohol abuse, what is *Zieve syndrome*?

A2. Zieve syndrome is jaundice, hemolytic anemia and hyperlipidemia/ hypercholesterolemia.

### 2. Veno occlusive disease (VOD) /Sinusoidal obstructive syndrome (SOS)

Q1. Liver transplantation may improve the clinical course of some patients with cystic fibrosis (CF). These LT-CF patients may develop VOD/SOS, but may also develop complications which are unique to LT-CF.

Give 2 unique GI complications of LT in CF.

A1.

- Secondary biliary cirrhosis → ↓ absorption of fat-soluble drugs; such as cyclosporin
- Distal intestinal obstruction syndrome (DIOS) (20%)

Q2. Veno-occlusive disease (aka sinusoidal obstruction syndrome [SOS]) occurs in up to 20% of HST patients, depending on the myloid-ablative conditioning used, and the presence of pre-existing liver disease. A clinical diagnosis may be made in the first three weeks after HCT. In difficult cases, WHVPG (wedge hepatic venous pressure gradient and liver biopsy may be necessary.

Give the *histological features* of SOS.

A2.
- Sinusoids
  - Dilated, disrupted
  - Fibrosis
  - Late collagenization
- Space of Disse
  - Extravasation of RBCs
- Hepatocytes
  - Zone 3 necrosis
  - Cell drop out
- Central vein (CV)
  - Subendothelial edema (CV remains potent)
  - Late colagenization

Unfortunately, the liver disease which led to the need for a liver transplantation (LT) may recur in the transplanted liver.

Q3. Give 5 types of liver disease which may *recur after LT* (liver transplantation)

A3.
- Infection
  - HBV*
  - HCV
- Immune
  - PBC
  - PSC
  - AIH
- Metabolic
  - NASH
- Toxins
  - ALD**

*Acquisition of HBV after LT does not alter 5 year survival rate , 25% redeveloping cirrhosis

**Depends of course if person begins drinking alcohol again

Abbreviations: AIH, autoimmune hepatitis; ALD, alcoholic liver disease; HBV, hepatitis B virus; HCV, hepatitis C virus ($99^{+}$ % recurrence); NASH, non-alcoholic lsteatohepatitis; PBC, primary biliary cirrhosis

Q4. What is the clinical course of *C. difficile in SOT* (solid organ transplantation)?

A4.
- Common
- May be clinically mild
- When severe, may be associated with
  - Megacolon
  - Death
- Poor response to antibiotics (only ~70%)

Q5. What is the benefit of probiotics for C. difficile infection in the immunosuppressed SOT patient?

A5. None. In fact beware, there may be an ↑ risk of yeast infection and dissemination!

Q6. Pancreatitis is common in the SOT setting (liver –Tx, 5%; Kidney – Tx, ~2%).

Give 7 common causes of this *post-SOT pancreatitis*.

A6.
- Infiltration
  - Malignancy
- Drug / toxins
  - Alcohol
  - Azathioprine
  - Steroids
  - Cyclosporin
  - Tacrolimus
- Cholelithiasis (perhaps because of precipitation of cyclosporin in bile, formimg the nidus for crystalization and stone formation)
- Surgical manipulation of pancreas

## 3. Liver failure

Q1. The commonest cause of death in adult-onset Still disease (A-OSD) (the adult form of juvenile RA) is liver failure. In the milder cases with hepatitis, the clinical presentation includes fever, sorethroath, weight loss, abdominal pain, jaundice, hepatosplenomegaly, ↑ ALT / AST.

Give the hepatic histological changes in *A-OSD*.

A1.

- Hepatitis
  - Interface
  - Lobular
- Lymphoplastic infiltration

## 4. NAFLD /NASH

Q1. The pathogenesis of the progression of NAFLD to NASH involves insulin resistance, as well as oxidative stress. There is evidence that Vitamin E (alpha tocopherol may benefit NASH.

Give the 10 benefits and AEs (adverse effects) of *TZD (pioglitazone)*.

| A1. Benefit | AEs |
|---|---|
| ↓ adipokinins | ↑ BMI |
| ↑ adiponection (a protector of the liver) | ↑ CV event |
| ↑ β oxidation | ↑ osteoporosis |
| ↓ TG, ↓ VLDL | ↑ bladder cancer |
| Converts "bad" into "good" fat | |
| ↓ insulin resistance | |

Q2. Patients with NAFLD may have elevated serum levels of ALT and AST. What level of these liver enzymes should signal the need to refer the patient for a *liver transplantation* (L-Tx)?

A2. No level! The decision to refer the NAFLD patient for L-Tx is based on the risk factors for progressing to NASH, and not on the level of their ALT or AST. In fact, ~ 60% of persons with NASH-cirrhosis have normal transaminases.

Q3. Bariatric surgery may improve NASH; how useful is *dieting* for persons with NASH?

A3. There is an inverse linear relationship between increasing weight loss and a decline in NAS (NAFLD activity score; even just a 5% loss of body weight has a clinically meaningful decline in NAS)

Q4. Does weight loss in NAFLD reduce mortality of this liver disease?

A4. Persons with NAFLD treated with weight loss have a reduced mortality rate from both cardiovascular as well as hepatic causes of death.

## 5. Acute and Chronic liver disease

Q1. What locations/ parts of the nervous system are affected by *hepatic encephalopathy* (HE)?

A1.
- Cortex
- Cerebellum
- Basal ganglia
- Spinal cord
- Peripheral nerves
- Muscles
- Hepatic histology shows
  - Normal histology, or
  - NAFLD, or
  - Mild portal cirrhosis

Q2. Mallory bodies (MB) are seen in alcoholic (ALD) as well as non-alcoholic liver disease (NAFLD). What are the *constituents of MB*?

A2. Mallory bodies arise from the accumulation of intermediated filaments.

Q3. Usually the ALT>AST in liver disease, However, the ALT is reduced and AST>ALT in ALD, NAFLD; Wilson disease or in association with a jejuno-ileal bypass, Why?

A3. ALT is reduced in ALD/NAFLD because of the effect of these two conditions on hepatic pyridoxal 5'-phosphate.

Q4. Give 8 factors which may explain the *inter-individual sensitivity to alcohol.*

A4.

- Varying levels of alcohol dehydrogenase (ADH), leading to higher levels of acetaldehyde.
- CYP2E1, leading to ↑ free radicals
- ↑ lipolysis, leading to ↑ synthesis of TG
- ↑ LPS (lipopolysaccharide) absorption
- ↑ TNF α (Kuppfer cells)
- ↑ oxidative damage
- ↑ peroxidative damage
- ↓ antioxidant protection
- Nutritional factors
- Possible autoimmune factors
- Drugs/ toxins
- Body iron stores
- α1, AT deficiency

Q5. We are taught to be non-judgemental in our

relationship with persons with alcoholism. Persons with ALD who meet a number of medical and social criteria may be offered a liver transplantation (L-Tx).

What is the alcohol *recidivism rate* after L-Tx for ALD?

A5. The alcohol recidivism rate after L-Tx for ALD is 10% to 15% at year 1 post L-Tx, and 25% to 50% at year 5.

Q6. Give five common *causes* of fatty liver other than ALD/NAFLD

A6.

- Metabolic
  - Metabolic syndrome
  - Abotalipoproteinemia
  - Wilson
  - Glycogen storage disease
- Infection
  - HCV
  - HIV
- Nutrition
  - TPN
  - Over/ undernutrition
- Surgery
  - Jejunoileal bypass
  - Gastroplasty

➢ Useful tid-bits
- A granuloma is comprised of a centre of epitheliod macrophages, surrounded by a rim of lymphocytes
- Peyer's patches are comprised of a collection of mucosal lymphoid cells
- Pus (purulent exudate) is comprised of a collection of neutrophils.

## 6. Cirrhosis

Q1. The patient with portal hypertension is examined, and does not have splenomegaly. Please give possible explanations.

A1.

- Asplenism
  - Congenital
  - Surgical removal
- Dextrocardia
- Multiple splenic infarcts (e.g. Sickle cell disease)
- Splenic vein thrombosis

## 7. Jaundice and Cholestasis

Q1. Which is the *better test* to assess the size of the liver in a patient with suggested cirrhosis, abdominal ultrasound with doppler, or transient elastography.

A1.

- Meta-analysis supports transient elastography to diagnose cirrhosis with a high diagnostic accuracy independent from the underlying liver disease (Friedrich-Rust, et al. *GE* 2008;134.960-974), and is not used to assess liver size.

➢ For a list of factors contributing to postoperative jaundice, please see Feldman M, et al. Sleisenger and Fordtran's Gastrointestinal and Liver Disease. 9$^{th}$ Edition. *Saunders/Elsevier* 2010, Table 35.7, page 583.

Q2. Give the typical histological changes seen on liver biopsy of *a jaundiced post-operative patient.*

A2. The typical histological changes seen on liver biopsy in the perioperative setting include:

- o Intrahepatic cholestasis
- o Kupffer cell erythrophagocytosis
- o Centrilobular congestion

Q3. The commonest cause of death in adult-onset Still disease (A-OSD) (the adult form of juvenile RA) is liver failure. In the milder cases with hepatitis, the clinical presentation includes fever, sorethroath, weight loss, abdominal pain, jaundice, hepatosplenomegaly, ↑ ALT / AST.

Give the *hepatic histological changes* in A-OSD.

A3.
- o Hepatitis
  - – Interface
  - – Lobular
- o Lymphoplastic infiltration

Q4. List 4 possible causes for failure to achieve pain relief after biliary sphincterotomy for presumed *sphincter of Oddi dysfunction (SOD).*

A4.
- ➢ Sphincter
  - o Inadequate initial sphincterotomy (remaining ↑ SOD pressure)
  - o Restenosis
- ➢ Pancreatitis
  - o Chronic pancreatitis with a normal pancreatogram
  - o Non-pancreaticobiliary pain (beware functional gastrointestinal disease)

Source*:* Feldman M, et al. *Saunders/Elsevier* 2006, page 1365.

Q5. What proportion of patients having a bone marrow transplant (BMT); (hematopoietic cell transplant) develop jaundice due to *GVHD* (graft-versus-host disease)?

A5. 20%; implication – don't assume that jaundice in BMT patients is related to GVHD.

Q6. In the context of cholestasis, what is *Stauffer-syndrome*?

A6. Stauffer syndrome is intrahepatic cholestasis and hepatosplenomegaly occurring as a paraneoplastic syndrome arising from lymphoma or renal cell carcinoma.

Q7. Give the performance characteristics for diagnostic *imaging studies* in cholestasis.

A7.

- Ultrasound
    - Gallbladder – sensitivity (sens) ~ 80%, specificity (spec) ~90%
    - Bile ducts, low sensitivity (sens) and specificity (spec)

| | Sens | Spec |
|---|---|---|
| - CT | 80% | 95% |
| - MRCP | 90% | 95% |
| - ERCP | 90% | 95% |
| - PTC | 99% | 95% |
| - EUS | 95% | 95% |

Q8. Give 5 conditions in which UDCA (*ursodeoxycholic acid*) is therapeutically beneficial.

A8.
- o PBC
- o Intrahepatic cholestasis
- o TPN-associated cholestasis
- o CF-associated cholestasis
- o Bone marrow-associated cholestasis
- o Prevention/reduction of formation of gallstones in persons undergoing bariatric surgery

*Note: Deduct marks for suggesting use of high dose UDCA in PSC

Q9. In most patients with viral hepatic, the liver is usually enlarged and tender whereas the spleen is enlarged and none tender. Which hepatic infection instead causes a large, tender spleen and non-tender hepatomegaly?

A9. EPV (Epstein Barr virus)

Q10. What is the clinical use of auscultating for a hepatic bruit or friction rub?

A10.
- o Hepatic arterial bruit
  - Alcoholic hepatitis
  - HCC (hepatocellular cancer)
  - Metastases
- o Venous hum
  - Portal hypertension(PHT, usually from cirrhosis, aka Cruveilhier-Bamgarten syndrome)
- o Venous hum plus hepatic arterial bruit (PHT+ alcoholic hepatitis, or PHT + HCC)
- o Rub + bruit
  - HCC
- o Friction rub
  - Infection in and around liver (e.g. gonococcal perihepatitis [Fitz-Hugh-Curtis syndrome])

Q11. Give the one cause of acute liver disease in which ascites commonly occurs.

A11. Budd Chiari syndrome

- Suspect infectious mononucleosis when both the liver and spleen are involved in and acute inflammatory process

Q12. Give the valve of the standard liver enzymes or liver function tests which lead to the suspicion of *Wilson disease*

A12.

- ↑↑ bilirubin, ↓ AP, ↑↑↑ bilirubin/ AP
- When diagnosing Wilson disease, remember that ceruloplasmin is an acute phase reactant, and that he urinary copper may be elevated in most forms of cholestatic liver disease.

Q13. Name three *liver tissue stains* for copper (Cu)

A13.

- Orcein, rubianic acid, rhodamine
- Because these are not sensitive, and in the presence of cholestasis are not specific, actual chemical analysis of the liver for Cu is advised.

Q14. Is it correct that KF *rings* are pathognomic for Wilson disease?

A14. Nope. KF rings may occur in any condition associated with chronic cholestasis.

Q15. What are the indications for *genetic testing* in the patient with suspected Wilson disease?

A15. None, this is because there are numerous genetic changes. Testing may be indicated after the diagnosis is made, in order to establish a pedigree.

Q16. What is the *recurrence* rate of symptomatic Wilson disease after L-Tx?

A16. Zero; it doesn't recur.

Q17. In the person with asymptomatic *iron overload* from HFE, what are the advantages of iron depletion by phlebotomy?

A17.

- ↓ hepatic fibrosis
- Possible ↓ in risk of HCC
- ↓ CHF/ arrhythmias in persons with excessive iron deposition in the heart (this risk is greater with cardiac iron overload associated with thalassemia rather than with hemochromatosis)

Q18. What is the prevalence of a symptomatic HFE?

A18. It depends: prevalence of the HFE genotype is 1/227, but only 28% of men and 1% of women with C282 Y develop symptoms. Studies are in progress to attempt to determine why there are so many "non-expressers" in HFE.

Q19. What is the *relationship* between liver iron concentration, and the extent of the abnormality in liver enzymes (LE)?

A19. The greater the abnormality in LE, the less likely is the diagnosis HFE.

Q20. What is the effect of alcohol intake on the *iron parameters* in HFE?

A20. Alcohol (ethanol) increases the serum concentration of ferritin and the hepatic RE cell content of iron.

Q21. What are thé characteristic of the *diabetes* which develops in HFE?

A21.

- Diabetes (DM) is not common in HFE, and if it occurs, there is usually cirrhosis present
- The DM is usually insulin resistant.

Q22. What is the risk of HFE in siblings or children of a person with HFE?

A22. The risk of HFE in the siblings of an HFE patient is 1.4, and in the HFE person's children, >1.20.

Q23. A person who is *C 282 Y* positive is diagnosed with HFE; in what partner will the phenotype be exposed?

A23. Non-expressors, 50% of females, 20% of males.

Q24. What is the use of measuring serum immunoglobulins in persons with liver disease?

A24. IgA, alcoholic liver disease
IgG, autoimmune liver disease
IgM, PBC

Q25. What is the use of *fiberscan* in PBC?

A25. PBC is a patchy disease of the small bile ducts, and there may be considerable sampling error in the demonstration of fibrosis/ nodular/ regeneration.

Q26. What is an *acidophil body*?

A26. The pink acidophil body represents a dying hepatocyte.

Q27. *Dupuytren contracture* (DC) is caused by thickening and flexure contraction of the palmar tendons, usually of the $4^{th}$ and $5^{th}$ digit (never the $1^{st}$ digit, i.e. thrumb). We all know that DC is associated with alcoholism (~40%) or alcoholic liver disease (~40%). Give 4 other GI or non-GI conditions are commonly associated with DC?

A27.
- Other GI conditions
  - Peptic ulcer disease
  - Cholecystitis
- Non GI conditions
  - Lung – tuberculosis
    – smokers
  - CNS – epilepsy
  - Endocrine – diabetic retinopathy

Science is work in progress – an evolution finding the truth

## 8. Hepatocellular Cancer (HCC)

Q1. What is the clinical use of auscultating *hepatic bruit or friction rub*?

A1.

- Hepatic arterial bruit
  - Alcoholic hepatitis
  - HCC (hepatocellular cancer)
  - Metastases
- Venous hum
  - Portal hypertension(PHT, usually from cirrhosis, aka Cruveilhier-Bamgarten syndrome)
- Venous hum plus hepatic arterial bruit (PHT+ alcoholic hepatitis, or PHT + HCC)
- Rub + bruit
  - HCC
- Rub and bruit + venous hum
  - Cirrhosis and HCC
- Friction rub
  - Infection in and around liver (e.g. gonococcal perihepatitis [Fitz-Hugh-Curtis syndrome])

"Only those who will risk going too far can possibly find out how far one can go"

T.S. Eliot

Q2. Give 10 *paraneoplastic syndromes* associated with HCC.

A2.

| | |
|---|---|
| ➢ CNS | ○ Neuropathy |
| ➢ Endocrine | ○ Sexual changes- isosexual precocity, gynecomastia, feminization |
| ➢ MSK | ○ Carcinoid syndrome |
| | ○ Hypercalcemia |
| | ○ Hypertrophic osteoarthropathy |
| | ○ Hypoglycemia |
| | ○ Osteoporosis |
| | ○ Polymyositis |
| | ○ Thyrotoxicosis |
| | ○ Thrombophlebitis migrans |
| ➢ CVS | ○ Systemic arterial hypertension |
| ➢ Skin | ○ Porphyria |
| ➢ GI | ○ Watery diarrhea syndrome |
| ➢ Hematology | ○ Polycythemia (erythrocytosis) |

Adapted from: Feldman M, et al. *Saunders/Elsevier* 2010, Table 94.2, page 1571.

Q3. Give 7 risk factors for *HCC in HBV*.

A3.

- Patient
  - Presence of cirrhosis
  - Young age of acquisition
  - Asian or African race
  - Male gender
  - Older age
  - Family history of HCC
  - Exposure to aflatoxin, alcohol, and tobacco
- Infection
  - Co-infection with HCV, HDV, and possibly HIV
  - Active replication of HBV
  - Genotype C

Q4. Give 7 risk factors for *HCC in HCV.*

A4.

- Patient
  - Alcohol drinking (heavy > 50 gm/d)
  - Male gender
  - Larger BMI
- Liver
  - Degree of hepatic fibrosis
- Infection
  - HBV co-infection
  - Older age of HCV onset and diagnosis
  - HIV co infection
  - Absence of previous HCV treatment
  - Long duration of active disease

Adapted from: El-serag HB. 2009 *ACG Annual Postgraduate Course*: 39-43.

Q5. Give 7 patient groups requiring *screening for HCC*.

A5.
- Hepatitis B carriers
    - Asian males >40
    - Asian females >50
    - Family history of HCC
    - African >20 years
    - All cirrhosis
- Non hepatitis B cirrhosis
    - Hepatitis C
    - Alcoholic cirrhosis
    - Hereditary hemochromatosis
    - Primary biliary cirrhosis
    - Possibly: alpha 1 antitrypsin, NASH, autoimmune

Source: El-serag HB. *2009 ACG Annual Postgraduate Course*: 39-43.

## 9. Liver granulomas

Q1. Give the mechanism of development of *hepatic granuloma*, and the histological changes.

A1. Lesions form and obliterate small portal veins and hepatic veins. This leads to ischemia, atrophy and then to nodular regenerative hyperplasia (NRH) comprised of:

- Multiple, monoacinar nodules resulting in nodular proliferation of hepatocytes (nodular transformation)
- The nodular proliferation of hepatocytes may compress the liver plates at the periphery of the nodules.
- No fibrous septa

Q2. NRH is associated with all the usual complications of portal hypertension.

What are the biochemical tests which reflect the functions of the liver, and outline the changes in the *liver function* test which occur in NRH.

A2. the functions of the liver are to synthesize proteins such as albumin and coagulation factors, and to excrete chemicals such as bilirubin and bile acids. Because of the regenerative hyperplasia of the hepatocyte, these hepatic functions are preserved despite the associated portal hypertension.

**10. Diagnostic Imaging**

Give the Distinguishing Diagnoses on Diagnostic Imaging

- Hemangioma vs Vascular tumor

| | Hemangioma | Vascular tumor |
|---|---|---|
| Ultrrasound | | |
| Mass hyperchoic | + | + |
| Hypogenic halo | - | + |
| RBC scan | | |
| Uptake early | - | + |
| Uptake late | + | |

- Cyst vs. cystic tumor

| | Cyst | Cystic Tumor |
|---|---|---|
| CT: enhancing rim | - | + |
| Doppler: internal blood flow | - | + |

- FNH, Adenoma, Fibrolamellar HCC

| | FNH | Hepatic adenoma | Fibrolamellar HCC |
|---|---|---|---|
| Enhancement | Homogenous | Heterogeneous | Homogeneous |
| Central stellate scar | + | - | + |
| Adenopathy, invasion of vessels | - | - | + |

- HCC vs Dysplastic Nodule

| | HCC | Dysplastic nodule |
|---|---|---|
| High-intensity-weighted mass | + | + |
| High intensity mass | + | - (remains isointense) |

- HCC, Lipoma and Hematoma

| | HCC | Lipoma | Hematoma |
|---|---|---|---|
| $T_{1/2}$ – weighted hyperintense mass | + | - | |
| Capsule | + | - | - |

- HCC vs hepatic metastases

| | HCC | Metastases |
|---|---|---|
| Multifocal | + | + |
| Dominant lesion | + | - |
| Hyperattenuation on early phase contrast enhancement | + | - |

- Intrahepatic cholangiocarcinoma (IHC)
    - HCC – hypervascular
    - Cystadenomas – cystic, lobular (septated)
    - Metastasis – cannot be distinguished from IHC

- Intrahepatic cholangiocarcinoma (IHC)
    - HCC – hypervascular
    - Cystadenomas – cystic, lobular (septated)
    - Metastasis – cannot be distinguished from IHC

- Biliary cystadenocarcinoma
    - Echinococcal cysts
        - Thin septae (not thick)
        - “daughter” cyst
        - Calcifications, fine

## Pancreas

Q1. In the context of a possible cholangiocarcinoma seen on diagnostic imaging, what is the *Mirizzi syndrome.*

A1. The Mirizzi syndrome is a stone in the cystic duct, which externally compresses the common bile duct (CBD), and looks like a CBD filing defect which could be easily confused to be a CBD tumor, such as cholangiocarcinoma.

Q2. Give the *Ranson prognostic criteria* for acute pancreatitis.

- On admission
    - Age (years) >55 >70
    - White blood cell count (cells/$mm^3$) >16, 000 >18, 000
    - Blood glucose (mg/dL) >200 >220
    - Lactate dehydrogenase (IU/L) >350 >400
    - Aspartate aminotransferase (IU/L) >250 >250

- During Initial 48 hours
    - Decrease in hematocrit (%) >10 >10
    - Increase in blood urea nitrogen (mg/dL) >5 >2
    - Calcium (mg/dL) <8 <8
    - $pO_2$ (mm Hg) <60 NA
    - Base deficit (mEq/L) >4 >5
    - Estimated fluid sequestration (L) >6 >4

Source:Quoted from original paper in Feldman M, et al. *Saunders/Elsevier* 2006, page 1241-1270.

Q3. In gallstone pancreatitis, give the explanation why there is first an elevation in serum ALT or AST, followed by ALP.

A3.
- Aminotransferases (ALT, AST) are released early from damaged hepatocytes.
- ALP is produced from the gallstone obstruction inducing the synthesis of this enzyme from the bile duct cells, so the process takes longer and ALP peaks later.

Q4. There are literally hundreds of *drugs* which may cause pancreatitis. Give drugs commonly seen being used in *GI patients* which are considered to have a moderately strong association with the development of pancreatitis.

A4.

| | |
|---|---|
| ➢ PUD | ○ Cimetidine<br>○ ASA<br>○ NSAIDs (e.g. sulindac) |
| ➢ Ascites | ○ Furosemide<br>○ Thiazides |
| ➢ IBD | ○ Azathioprine, 6-MP<br>○ Sulfasalazine<br>○ Metronidazole |
| ➢ Tropical sprue | ○ Tetracycline |

"Discipline is the bridge between goals and accomplishments"

Jim Rohn

## 1. Abdominal X-ray

Q1. Give 7 causes of *calcification* on abdominal X – ray.

A1.
- Lumen of bowel - Fecoliths
- UEIN - Phleboliths
- Nodes - Calcified lymph nodes
- Stones - Calculi-renal, gall bladder, prostatic
- Glands - Calcified pancreas, adrenal, liver (see below), kidney, aorta, psoas muscle, costal cartilage
- Tumor - Calcified tumor-dermoid, fibroid
- Fetus
- Abdominal wall - Calcification in abdominal wall, e.g. cysticerci
- Foreign body on abdominal wall

Adapted from: Burton JL. *Churchill Livingstone* 1971, page 49.

Q2. Give 7 causes of radiological *hepatic calcification*

A2.
- Infection
  - Hydatid cysts
  - Amoebic abscess
  - TB
  - Histoplasmosis
  - Gumma
  - Brucellosis
- Tumor
  - Hepatoma (HCC)
- Veins
  - Hemangioma
- Intrahepatic bile ducts
  - Calculi

Adapted from: Burton JL. *Churchill Livingstone* 1971, page 49.

Q3. Metastases to the lung are usually seen as a few large deposits. From what primary tumors are the *metastases to the lung* usually multiple and small?

A3. Lung metastasis from primary cancers of
- Bronchus
- Stomach

Q4. What is the difference between *mottling and miliary mottling* on a chest X-ray?

A4.
- Mottling is multiple, discrete semi-confluent shadows, < 5 mm.
- Military mottling is multiple, discrete, bilateral shadows, < 2 mm.

## 2. Cysts

Q1. IPMN (intraductal papillary mucinous neoplasm) may occur in the MD (main pancreatic duct; MD-IPMN) or BD (branch duct; BD-IPMN).

Give the *Sendi guidelines* which help to distinguish low from high risk of malignancy developing in IPMN, and therefore the criteria for surgical resection.

A1.
- Resect
  - All MD-IPMN
  - BD-IPMN
    - > 3 cm
    - Symptoms ("…pain is a predictor of underlying malignancy" [from IPMN] (Spiegel, BMR, et al. *Slack Incorporated* 2011, page 145).
  - MD- / BD-IPMN with nodules or thickening on EUS CEA > 192

Q2. A high *amylase* concentration in the aspirated mucus from an IPMN *does not fit* with Sendi guidelines / or resection of the tumor. Please explain why.

A2.
- An ↑ amylase in the aspirated fluid in IPMN means that the duct communicates with the main pancreatic duct, but the lesion could be BD or MD.
- MD-IPMN must be resected because of its high malignant potential, but finding ↑ amylase in fluid means this could be MD- or BD-IPMN.
- If the IPMN < 3 cm, no symptoms, no nodules or thickening, and CEA < 192, then surveillance could be offered q 6-12 months (CT, MRI / MRCP, EUS)

Q3. What is the pathological composition of "*pus*".

A3.
- Pus, or mucopurulent material, is comprised of mucus mixed with PMNs

**3. VIPoma**

Q1.Give the clinical and laboratory features of *VIPoma syndrome*.

A1.
- Diarrhea
  - Secretory
  - Volume depletion
- Weight loss
- Abdominal pain
- Flushing
- Laboratory Findings
  - ↓ $K^+$, $Cl^-$
  - ↑ $Ca^{2+}$, blood sugar

Abbreviations: VIPoma, vasoactive intestinal peptide secreting pancreatic endocrine tumor.

Adapted from: Feldman M, et al. *Saunders/Elsevier* 2010, Table 32-8, page 509.

### 4. Somatostatinoma

Q1. The Somatostatinoma Syndrome is complished by diarrhea, weight loss, diabetes, and gallstones; hypochlorhydria may also be a feature. Give the pathophysiological basis of the clinical features, based on the actions of somatostatin (SS-14 and SS-28)

A1.

- Diarrhea
  - ↓ pancreatic secretion
  - ↓ lipid digestion
  - ↓ lipid absorption
- Weight loss
  - Steatorrhea (see above)
- Diabetes
  - ↓ insulin release
- Gallbladder disease
  - ↓ gallbladder motility → ↑ biliary sludge / stones
- Hypochlorhydria
  - ↓ gastric acid secretion

Q2. About 10% of patients with leukemia have involvement of GI tract, relating to infiltration of leukemia cells into the GI tract, associated immunodeficiency, coagulation defects, drug toxicity, and complications associated with bone marrow transplantation (see Feldman M, et al. *Saunders/Elsevier* 2010; Table 35.3, page 566)

In the patient with acute or chronic leukemia who presents with an *acute abdomen*, give 4 of the most common causes, which are related to the leukemia.

A2.
- Acute appendicits
- Intra-abdominal abscess
- Perforation
- Necrotizing enterocolitis (ileum and cecum)
- Typhlitis (inflammation of cecum, often in the presence of neutropenia)

*Note:

- The sensitivity of these tests to detect insulinoma is generally 10% to 20% lower
- The sensitivity of these to detect hepatic metastases arising from pancreatic endocrine tumors is generally > 20% higher

Q3. In the context of glucagonoma, what other conditions cause *necrolytic migratory erythema* (NME) and hyperglucagonemia.

A3.
- ➢ Conditions associated with NME
  - Small intestine
    - IBD
    - Celiac disease
    - Short bowel syndrome
    - Nutritional deficiency
  - Liver
    - Cirrhosis
    - HBV infection
  - Stomach
    - ZES
- ➢ Conditions associated with hyperglucagonemia

- Small bowel
  - Celiac disease
- Liver
  - Cirrhosis
- Pancreas
  - Acute pancreatitis
- Kidney
  - Chronic renal failure
- Endocrine
  - Diabetic ketoacidosis
  - Starvation
  - Acromegaly
  - Hypercorticism
- Trauma
  - Burns
  - Sepsis
- Drugs
  - Danazol
- Familial

## 5. Diagnostic Imaging

Give the Distinguishing Diagnoses on Diagnostic Imaging

- Solid, hypoechoic pancreatic mass(es)
  - Adenocarcinoma
  - Matastases
  - Islet cell tumors
  - Lymphoma
  - Focal pancreatitis

- Islet cell tumor (ICT) metastasis to livers vs. hepatic hemangioma on ultrasound

| | Echogenic | Posterior Acoustic Shadowing |
|---|---|---|
| Hemangioma | + | - |
| ICT | + | + |

- Ductal Adenocarcinoma vs. Islet Cell Tumors

| Features | Ductal Adenocarcinoma | Islet cell Tumor |
|---|---|---|
| Size | ≤ 4 cm | 0.5 mm to 100 mm |
| Vascularity | ↓ | ↑ |
| Vascular Encasement | ++++ | + |
| Calcification | + | ++++ |
| Duct dilation | ++++ | + |

- Primary lymphoma, ductal adenocarcinoma, non-functioning ICT

| | Primary Lymphoma | Ductal Adeno-carcinoma | Non-functioning ICT |
|---|---|---|---|
| Circumscribed | + | - | |
| Vascular encasement | - | + | |
| Pancreatic / Bile duct obstruction | - | + | |
| Homogeneous | + | | - |
| Hyper-enhancement | + | - | + |
| Calcification | - | | + |

 

## Gallbladder and Biliary Tree

### 1. Gallstone

Q1. Give 3 causes of *pneumobilia*.

A1.
- Sphicterotomy
- Gallstone ileus
- Chlostridium perfringens infection (gas-forming organism)

Q2. Give the likely *sites* of obstruction in *gallstone ileus*, depending on the size of gallstone.

A2.
- Ileocecal valve, > 2 cm
- Sigmoid colon, > 2.5 cm
- "rolling obstruction" – the site of the mechanical obstruction moves ("rolls") distally as the gallstone passes along the small and large intestines.

Q3. About 10% of pregnant woman develop gallstones, and 1% have symptomatic cholelithiasis. When should *cholecystectomy* be performed in a pregnant woman for symptomatic biliary colic or gallstone pancreatitis?

A3.
- It is recommended that a woman with symptomatic gallstones should have a laparoscopic cholecystectomy, and not be followed "expectantly".
- This "do-surgery-now" approach is rationalized by the high morbidity for the mother and the fetus if there is a recurrent episode of cholecystitis / pancreatitis.
- Ideally perform cholecystectomy in $T_2$, because

surgery in $T_1$ may lead to fetal mortality, and during $T_3$ surgery may lead to premature delivery.

Q4. In the presence of obstructive jaundice, a *palpable gallbladder* is not due to cholelithiasis. What are the *exceptions* to this clinical “rule”?

A4. Stones in the cystic duct, or Hartmann’s pouch.

## 2. Splenomegaly

Q1. *Splenomegaly accompanies hepatomegaly* in persons with portal hypertension. What are the exceptions to this clinical “rule”?

A1.
- Congenital asplenia
- Post-surgical asplenia
- Splenic vein thrombosis
- Multiple splenic vein infarctions

Q2. Percussion in *Traub’s space* is not specific for splenomegaly. What other conditions cause dullness here?

A2.
- Left pleural effusion
- Large pericardial effusion
- Massive cardiomegaly
- Stomach full of food
- Splenic flexure of colon full of feces
- Enlarged left kidney

### 3. Biliary Tree

Q1. Define "*Choledochal cyst*", and give examples of the common types.

A1. Definition: Choledochal cysts are congenital "segmental dilations of the biliary tree that can lead to …complications, including structures, recurrent pancreatitis, and cholangiocarcinoma" [30%] (Spiegel, BMR, et al. *Slack Incorporated* 2011, page 67).

- Types I, CBD diffusely enlarged, with tapered ends ("fusiform")
- Type II, CBD diverticula
- Type III, Dilation of intraduodenal portion of CBD (aka "choledochcele")
- Type IV, Multiple intra- and extra-hepatic cysts of the bile ducts
- Type V, Diffuse intrahepatic cysts

➢ Usual treatment
- Surgery – I, II
- Sphincterotomy – III

Q2. In the context of cholangiohepatitis, give the Reynold's Pentad modification of *Charcot's Triad*.

A2.

➢ Charcot's Triad (CT)
- RUQ pain
- Jaundice
- Fever

➢ Reynold's Pentad: CT plus
- Hypotension
- Altered mental status

## 4. Diagnostic Imaging

Give the Distinguishing Diagnoses on Diagnostic Imaging

- Intrahepatic Cholangiocarcinoma (CC)
    - Cannot be distinguished from metastatic lesions to liver
    - HCC is hypervascular, CC is not
    - Biliary cystadenoma
- Porcelain gallbladder
    - "clean" posterior acoustic shadowing: single, thin echogenic (white) line
- Emphasematous gallbladder
    - "dirty" posterior shadowing
- Gallbladder filled with stones
    - "wall-echo-shadow": echogenic line
    - Lucency
    - Echogenic line
- Cholelithiasis
    - "clean" posterior shadowing plus echogenic arc acoustic
- Milk of calcium bile
    - Gallbladder and cystic duct are opaque on abdominal plain radiograph, and hyperattenuated (white) on unenhanced CT
- Distinguishing features on ultrasound:

| | Stones | Sludge | Polyp / Tumor |
|---|---|---|---|
| "clean" posterior acoustic shadowing | + | - | - |
| Mobility | + | + | - |
| Internal blood flow | - | - | + |

## Nutrition

### 1. Refeeding syndrome

Q1. Define the "*refeeding syndrome*", and outline its pathophysiological basis.

A1.
- If glucose is fed rapidly, insulin is released, phosphate is rapidly taken up into cells, and the serum $PO_4^-$ falls
  - The complications which develop include:
    - Neurological (seizures, paresthesias, hyperosmolar coma) and cardiovascular (CCF, death)
    - GI – diarrhea
    - RBC fail to release $O_2$ normally → VT (ventricular tachycardia)
    - Acute thiamine deficiency (wet beriberi) may develop on the initiation of peripheral as well as total parenteral nutrition
- The cells in PEM are depleted of $K^+$ & $Mg^{2+}$, and refeeding with glucose/ AAs shifts these back into cells, and may lead to serious cardiovascular adverse effects
- In order for hypocalcemia to be corrected, it is necessary to correct any associated body depletion of $Mg^{2+}$ (best assessed from urinary levels after IV infusion rather than from serum concentrations)
- Predigested monomeric or oligomeric elemental or semi-elemental diets are not superior to polymeric diets or whole food

Q2. In the context of gastrointestinal diseases, give the major complications arising from *deficiencies* of 6 of the following *micronutrients and vitamins:*

A2.
- Copper – anemia, altered taste
- Iodine – hypothyroidism
- Manganese – thin, light hair
- Selenium – myositis, cardiomyopathy, collagen vascular disease
- Zinc – acrodermatitis enterohepatica, impaired taste,

glucose intolerance, slow wound healing, alopecia, depression, diarrhea

- Chromium – glucose intolerance
- Thiamine (B1) – beriberi, Wernicke encephalopathy, polyneuritis, anorexia, anemia, ataxia
- Riboflavin – sore mouth & lips, swollen tongue, photophobia
- Niacin – pellagra – glossitis, dermatitis, mental confusion
- Pantothenic acid – poor wound healing

## 2. Obesity

Q1. Give 3 mechanisms explaining alterations in *serum vitamin levels in obesity*.

A1.
- ↓ intake
- ↓ transport proteins (chronic inflammation in obesity → ↑ pro-inflammatory cytokines
- ↑ turnover
- Shift in tissue distribution

Q2. Give 7 symptoms/ signs of *protein/ calorie malnutrition* (PCM) which may occur in obesity.

A2.
- General
  - Fatigue
  - Weakness
- Hair
  - Brittle
  - Loss of hair
  - Altered colour
- Skin
  - Edema
  - Pressure sores
  - Dry/ scaly skin
  - Slow healing
- CVS
  - Tachycardia

# Hematology

## 1. Myeloid disorders

Q1. What are the "*chronic myeloid disorders*"?

A1.
- Chronic myeloid leukemia
- Myelodysplastic syndrome
- Atypical chronic myeloid disorder
- Chronic myeloproliferative disease
  - Polycythamia vera
  - Myelofibrosis with myeloid metaplasia
  - Essential thrombocythemia
  - Agnogenic myeloid metaplasia
  - Post-polycythemic myeloid metaplasia
  - Post-thrombocythemic myeloid metaplasia

Source: Baliga RR. *Saunders/Elsevier* 2007, page 317.

Q2. What is the difference between "*myeloid metaplasia*" and "*extramedullary hematopoiesis*"?

A2. None: they both represent ectopic hematopoietic activity, usually in liver and spleen, and may not be associated with myelofibrosis (bone marrow fibrosis).

Q3. OK. What is "*myelofibrosis with myeloid metaplasia*"?

A3. By convention, is called idiopathic myelofibrosis

Source: Baliga RR. *Saunders/Elsevier* 2007, page 317.

**2. Purpura**

Q1. In the setting of a patient with purpura, what is *Moschcowitz's syndrome*?

A1.
- Speak English. Moschcowitz's syndrome is simply TTP (thrombotic thrombocytopenic purpura), an acute disorder characterized by:
  - Thrombocytpenic purpura
  - Microangiopathic haemolytic anemia
  - Transient and fluctuating neurological features
  - Fever
  - Renal impairment

Source: Baliga RR. *Saunders/Elsevier* 2007, page 391.

"You gain strength, courage and confidence by every experience in which you really stop to look fear in the face"

Eleanor Roosevelt

## Nephrology

### 1. Hypertension

Q1. Differentiate between *Pseudohypertension* and Pseudohypotension

A1.
- Pseudohypertension – Artery can be palpated when a blood pressure cuff is inflated to the point of obliterating the radial pulse, and the artery is still palpated as a firm tube in the absence of a pulse (Osler's maneuver).
  - Positive Osler's sign, indicating the presence of arterosclerosis, and both SBP and DBP be overestimated.
- Pseudohypotension – in conditions of high peripheral vascular resistance such as shock, Korotkoff sounds are difficult to use to measure accurately systolic or diastolic pressure.

Source: Mangione S. *Hanley & Belfus* 2000, pages 28 and 29.

Q2. In primary hyperaldosteronism, what are the effects of variations in the intake of salt (NaCl) on aldosterone and rennin?

A2.
- High salt intake – no effect on aldosterone
- Low salt intake – no effect on renin

## 2. Hypovolemia

Q1. What's the difference between *hypovolemia* (volume depletion) and *dehydration*.

A1.
- Hypovolemia; volume depletion is the loss of extracellular $Na^+$ from the GI tract or kidneys, leading to an increase in the serum urea nitrogen-to-creatinine, corrected by the rapid IV infusion of 0.9% "normal" saline to correct and associate hemodynamic instability.

- Dehydration is the loss of intracellular water, leading tc rise in serum $Na^+$ and plasma osmolality, corrected by the slow IV infusion of 5% D/W

Abbreviations: HE: Hypovolemia-Extracellular; DI: dehydration-intracellular)

> Some people are in their own jail
>
> *Anonymous*

## Respirology

### 1. Asthma

Q1. In the context of the patient with asthma, what is "*Loeffler's syndrome*"?

A.
- o Loeffler syndrome is comprised of
  - Asthma (airway reactivity)
  - Fever
  - Eosinophilia
  - Abnormal chest X-ray (transient, migratory pneumonitis; remember that persons with uncomplicated asthma will have a normal chest X-ray

- o Loeffler syndrome may be associated with
  - Polyartheritis
  - Allergic asthma
  - Allergic skin disease
  - Infections: mycoses, parasites
  - Drugs (e.g. Sulfa's, penicillin)

### 2. Breath sounds, signs

Q1. Are *breath sounds* reduced when ausculated over a *pleural effusion*?

A1. It depends.
- o Above the effusion-normal
- o At the margin of the effusion-increased
- o Over the rest of the effusion-reduced

Source: Mangione S. *Hanley & Belfus* 2000, page 305.

Q2. Does pneumonia increase or decrease *tactile vocal fremitus* (TVF)?

A2. It depends in bronchopneumonia (involving bronchi and alveoli, often from H. Influenza, with bronchial mucus plugs), ↑ in alveolar pneumonia (infection in alveoli but bronchial tree leaves bronchi pattern; the infectious fluid in the alveoli plus the air in the bronchi make the TVF increase.

Source: Mangione S. *Hanley & Belfus* 2000, page 288.

Q3. What is the effect of coughing on *expiratory crackles*?

A3. Obstructive disease, decreased course expiratory crackles restrictive disease, no change with coughing.

Source: Mangione S. *Hanley & Belfus* 2000, page 315.

Q4. Are late inspiratory crackles common in all types of intestinal lung disease?

A4. Common in Idioathic Pulmonary Fibrosis (IPF) or Asbestosis (60%), but uncommon in sarcoidosis (18%; upper lobe and peribronchial fibrosis, vs lower lobe and subpleural fibrosis in IPF).

Source: Mangione S. *Hanley & Belfus* 2000, page 317.

"The price of anything is the amount of life you exchange for it"

Henry David Thoreau

Q5. Can you distinguish a *pleural rub* from a *crackle*, a *wheeze* and a *pericardial rub*?

A5.
- A pleural rub
  - Present during both inspiration and expiration (never present only in expiration)
  - Does not change with coughing
  - Long, louder, lower-pitched than crackle
  - May be palpable

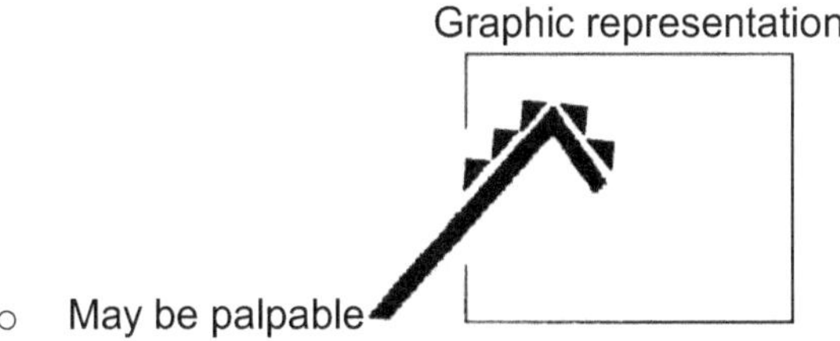


- A wheeze
  - Usually occur in expiration only, whereas rubs are usually heard in both inspiration and expiration, or just in inspiration, but never only in expiration.

- A pericardial rub
  - If the rub persists when the breath is held, then (dah!) it is more likely a pericardial than a pleural rub.

Source: Mangione S. *Hanley & Belfus* 2000, pages 310, 328 and 329.

Q6. How can you differentiate between *chronic bronchitis or asthma* versus *emphysema* by listening to the patient's breath sounds heard at the mouth (BSM) with the unaided ear, i.e. without using a stethoscope?

A6. In chronic bronchitis and asthma, there is a positive relation between the loudness of BSM and the $FEV_1$, or PEFR (peaked expiratory flow rate), whereas in asthma, BSM, becomes softer as airflow obstruction worsens. Thus, the intensity of BSM is not increased in all persons with COPD.

Source: Mangione S. *Hanley & Belfus* 2000, page 304.

Q7. During auscultation of the chest, if you hear *crackles or rhonchi*, do you ask the patient to cough?

A7. Why not! Coughing clears the crackles and rhonchi of airflow obstruction caused by extra sounds at air-fluid interfaces of medium-to-large airways.

Q8. What is the cause of a *clicking sound* which is synchronous with systole?

A8. Left – side pneumothorax

**3. Breathing**

Q1. What is *respiratory alternans* (aka paradoxical respiration, or abdominal paradox?

A1. Normally with inspiration both chest and abdominal wall rises. With muscular weakness and fatigue, the abdominal wall does not rise.

Q2. How does "*Biot breathing*" differ from *Cheyne – Stoke breathing*?

A2.
- Short periods of irregular breathing (varying rate and depth), followed by periods of apnea
- Usually seen in association with meningitis
- Biot breathing lacks the waxing and waning of Cheyne- Stokes breathing

Q3. How can you suspect if a person's dyspnea is on a *hysterical basis*?

A3. The breathing is deep, and the person holds their breath after about every six breaths.

Q4. In the persons with smoker's face and nicotine staining of fingers, pursed lips and using the accessory muscles of expiration (intercostals muscles), what is *Dahl sign*?

A4. Patches of hyperpigmented calluses above both knees from chronic pressure of the elbows on the skin of the legs resulting from sitting up and leaning forward to breath better (orthopnea), placing the elbows near the knees and fixing the position of the shoulder and the neck muscles to improve the contractility of the accessory muscles and improving basilar perfusion and lung mechanics.

Source: Mangione S. *Hanley & Belfus*, 2000, pages 277 and 280.

Q5. In what cause of *bronchopneumonia* is bronchial breathing as well as other physical findings usually absent, or minimal?

A5. Viral bronchopneumonia

### 4. Bronchiectasis

Q1. When *bronchiectasis* is caused by fibrosis from previous TB, in which lobes does the recurrent pneumonia usually occur?

A1. Upper lobes

Q2. Your patient has rhonchi and prolonged expiration, and you suspect bronchitis, but the chest X-ray is abnormal. What conditions are likely associated with her/ his *bronchitis*?

A2.
- Emphysema
- Bronchiectasis
- Pleural thickening

### 5. Chest X-ray

The "ABCs" of *Reading a Chest X-Ray*

**A** – airway (midline, no obvious deformities, no paratracheal masses).

**B** – bones and soft tissue (no fractures, subcutaneous emphysema).

**C** – cardiac size, silhouette, and retrocardiac density normal.

**D** – diaphragms (right above left by 1cm to 3cm, costophrenic angles sharp, diaphragmatic contrast with lung sharp).

**E** – equal volume 9count ribs, look for mediastinal shift).

**F** – fine detail (pleura and lung parenchyma).

**G** – gastric bubble (above the air bubble one shouldn't see an opacity of any more than 0.5cm width).

**H** – hilum (left normally above right by up to 3cm,

no larger than a thumb), hardware (in the intensive care unit: endotracheal tube, central venous catheters).

Source: Talley NJ, et al. *Maclennan & Petty Pty Limited* 2003, page 132.

Q1. Give the most common causes of *ring shadows* (small translucent areas with white margins) seen on chest X-ray.

A1.
- Bullae
- Cavities
- Cysts
- Localized pneumothorax

Q2. From a chest X-ray, how can you distinguish between the *homogeneous opacity* caused by a collapsed basal segment of the lung, and the heart border?

A2.
- The border of a collapsed segment may be sharp and straight
- The heart border follows a straight line

Q3. Under what circumstances does *pleural thickening become calcified*?

A3. Pleural thickening becomes calcified when there is associated serous or purulent effusion.

Q4. Under what circumstances is a haze, *homogenous opacity* on chest X-ray have a well-defined border?

A4. When it is due to collapse, rather than pleural thickening.

Q5. In the context of a pleural effusion seen on a lateral chest X-ray, what is "*Ellis S-shaped line*"?

A5. Ellis's S-shaped line is an S-shaped line seen in the axilla of a patient with an effusion which is encapsulated or associated with air.

Q6. In the context of an abnormal chest X-ray in a child, what is *Harrison sulcus*, and what are its causes?

A6.
- o Definition – Harrison's sulcus a groove which is directed down wards and outwards over the anterior chest wall
- o Causes
  - Rickets
  - Chronic chest infection

**6. Clubbing**

Q1. From the physical examination, what will suggest that the person's clubbing is the familial congenital form?

A1.
- o The person's heritage is often African
- o All the signs of clubbing; the loss of the subungual angle is common, but the presence of ballottement is less 50.

Q2. Other than form the family history, how can you distinguish familial from *non-familial clubbing*.

A2. Familial clubbing is
- o Asymmetrical
- o Increases with ageing

Q3. What is the cause of *unilateral clubbing of the right hand*?

A3. Aneurysm of the thoracic aorta

Q4. Under what circumstances is *clubbing* of the digits *painful*?

A4. When digital clubbing is associated with periostosis, periosteal formation of new bone, and hypertrophy (hypertrophic pulmonary osteoarthropathy, [HPO], aka Marie-Bamberger syndrome)

- The diagnosis of HPO is may be suspected clinically, but is confirmed by the radiological demonstration of periostosis.

Q5. Examine the dorsal portion of the fingers for *bulimia*.

A5. Abrasions, excoriations or calluses suggest chronic trauma on the fingers against the teeth as the sufferer repeatedly attempts to induce vomiting.

Q6. In the context of clubbing and bone pain as well as tenderness, what other physical signs suggest *hypertrophic pulmonary osteoarthropathy* (HPO)?

A6.

- Pretibial skin
    - Shiny
    - Warm
    - Red
    - Thickened
    - Sweating
- Hands and feet
    - Sweating
    - Warmth
    - Paresthesias
    - Clubbing, but note: not always associated with clubbing

- Systemic
  - Sweating
  - Warmth
  - Paresthesias

- Joints
  - Symmetrical
  - Arthritis-like changes in wrists, elbows, knees, ankles

- Subcutaneous tissue – coarsening in
  - Hands
  - Feet
  - Face

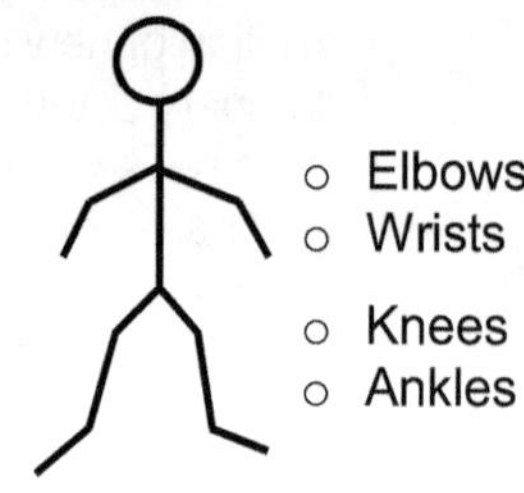

- Elbows
- Wrists
- Knees
- Ankles

- Causes
  - Lung
    - Bronchogenic cancer
    - Metastatic lung cancer
    - Mesothelioma
    - Bronchiectasis
    - Lung abscess
    - Chronic empyema
    - Cystic fibrosis - Note: HPO almost never occurs with pulmonary interstitial fibrosis
  - CVS
    - Infected aortic bypass graft
  - Liver
    - Cirrhosis

- Clinical course
  - HPO often resolves with cure of associated condition

Q7. What is hypertrophic pulmonary osteoarthropathy?

A7.
- Hypertrophic pulmonary osteoarthropathy is digital clubbing with periostosis (*Marie-Bamberger syndrome*)
- A systemic disorder of bones, joints, and soft tissues most commonly associated with an intrathoracic neoplasm (usually bronchogenic carcinoma but also lymphomas and metastatic cancers).
- Periosteal new-bone proliferation that accompanies digital clubbing, especially prominent in the long bones of the extremities.
- Other features of symmetric arthritis-like changes in one or more joints (ankles, knees, wrists, and elbows); coarsening of the subcutaneous tissue in the distal portions of arms and legs (and occasionally the face); neurovascular changes in hands and feet (with chronic erythema, paresthesias, and increased sweating).
- Associations may be seen in
  - Cystic fibrosis,
  - Brochiectasis,
  - Chronic empyema,
  - Lung abscesses (all typically associated with clubbing),
  - Pulmonary interstitial fibrosis

Source: Mangione S. *Hanley & Belfus* 2000, page 485.

**7. Lung collapse**

Q1. In the setting of the patient with a lung collapse, what is *Brock syndrome*?

A1. Brock syndrome is lung collapse due to compression of the right middle lobe bronchus by an enlarged lymph node, often from TB.

Source: Baliga RR. *Saunders/Elsevier* 2007, page 292.

Q2. Why may the middle lobe collapse and disappear in some persons suffering from a *pulmonary infarction*?

A2.
- o The right middle bronchus may collapse, the middle lobe may collapse, and retract towards the hilum
- o The remaining normal lung lobes may dilate (compensatory emphysema) and obscure the collapsed middle lobe.

**8. COPD**

Q1. Is *Campbell sign* specific for COPD?

A1. Tracheal descent with inspiration ("tracheal tug", aka Campbell's sign) is caused by any cause of chronic airflow obstruction, and not just COPD.

Source: Mangione S. *Hanley & Belfus* 2000, page 287.

Q2. Under what conditions does the auscultation of *vesicular breath sounds* not signify reduced air flow (e.g. in COPD)?

A2.
- o Normal thickness of the chest wall
- o Normal pleura (no fluid or air)
- o Normal function of respiratory muscles
- o Reduced/distant breath sounds suggest COPD, as also do vesicular breath sounds. Breath sounds of normal intensity mean that the FEV1 is normal or near normal.
- o Ausculation of the breath sound intensity (BSI) at the bedside (reduced intensity) correlates with FEV1, FEV1/FVC, and distribution of ventilation – a poor person's pulmonary function test – because of air-trapping and destruction of lung parenchyma in COPD

- In COPD (asthma, chronic bronchitis), the intensity of breath sounds heard at the mouth without the use of a strethoscope increases: with airway obstruction, intensity at mouth increases, over the chest diseases.

Source: Mangione S. *Hanley & Belfus* 2000, page 302.

## 9. Cyanosis

Q1. From inspection of the patient, how can you distinguish between *cyanosis and met-/ sulphemoglobinemia*?

A1. Persons with an excess of these abnormal hemoglobins do not have dyspnea.

## 10. Pulmonary function test (PFT)

Q1. How can you estimate the value of $FEV_1/FVC$ with your stethoscope? (!)

A1. Auscultate over sternal notch and time how long it takes the patient to take a deep breath and blow out hard. This gives the forced-expiratory time ($FET_0$).

| $FET_0$ | $FEV_1/FVC$ |
|---|---|
| >6 sec | ≤ 40% |
| <5 sec | > 60% |

Source: Mangione S. *Hanley & Belfus* 2000, page 304.

**11. Sarcoidosis**

Q1. What are the skin manifestations of *sarcoidosis*?

A1.
- Small, non-scaling, skin-coloured, dome-shaped papules, usually on face and neck
- If lesions coalesce, nodules and plaque form on the trunk and extremities

Source: Baliga RR. *Saunders/Elsevier* 2007, page 437.

**12. Deep vein Thrombosis (DVT)**

Q. In the context of deep vein thrombosis (DVT), what is *Virchow triad*?

A.
- Damage to the vessel wall
  - Trauma
  - Hypoxic blood
  - Drugs
  - Infection
  - Cholesterol
- ↓ blood flow
- ↑ blood coagulability

Source: Baliga RR. *Saunders/Elsevier* 2007, pages 100 and 101.

."Go confidently in the direction of your dreams. Live the life you have imagined"

Henry David Thoreau

## Rheumatology

### 1. Ankylosing spondilitis

Q1. In the context of ankylosing spondilitis, what is the normal chest expansion, and what is the *Schober test*?

A1.
- Normal chest expansion is 5 cm (2")
- Schober test – 10 cm. above the dimples of venus, flex forward maximally, the extension should by 5 cm (10cm → 15cm).

### 2. Calf

Q1. In the context of redness and swelling of the calf of one leg, what is the "*crescent sign*", and what diagnosis does it suggest?

A1. If there is crescent-shaped bruising of the calf from the medial to the lateral malleolus, they likely have pseudothrombophlebitis from a ruptured cyst.

### 3. Hip

Q1. In the context of a screening physical examination for hip disease, what is the *FABER maneuver*?

A1. The FABER maneuver is the movement of the hip so that it is Flexed, ABducted, and Externally Rotated. The lateral aspect of the leg should then be able to lay.

**4. Lyme disease**

Q1. While on a camping trip in Europe, a gentleman develops an annular rash. He returns home to North Overshore, and six weeks later he develops a painful knee joint and a unilateral facial nerve (CN VII) palsy. What is the likely etiology?

A1.
- o Lyme disease, and the confirmatory test is an antibody titre against *Borrelia burgdorferi*.

**5. Marfan syndrome**

Q1. How is the diagnosis for *Marfan syndrome* made?

A1.
- o With family history: features from 2 systems
- o Without a family history
  - Skeletal features (including pectus carinatum or excavatum, reduced lower upper-lower segment ratio, arm-span-to-height ratio > 1.05, scoliosis and reduced elbow extension
  - Involvement of at least two other systems and one of the major criteria
  - Ectopia lentis
  - Dilation of the aortic root or aortic dissection
  - Lumbosacral dural ectasia by CT or MRI

Q2. The skeletal phenotype of homocystinuria is similar to Marfan syndrome. How are the two distinguished on physical examination.

A2.
- o In homocystinuria the lens is dislocated downwards (and there is homocystine in the urine).

Source: Baliga RR. *Saunders/Elsevier* 2007, page 581.

## 6. Rheumatioid arthritis

Q1. What causes *arthritis plus nodules*?

A1.
- Rheumatoid arthritis
- Systemic lupus erythematosus (rare)
- Rheumatic fever (Jaccoud's arthritis) (very rare)
- Granulomas- e.g. sarcoid (very rare)

Source: Talley NJ, et al. *Maclennan & Petty Pty Limited* 2003, page 269.

Q2. A nodule is palpated at the extensor surface of the elbow. How can you differentiate between a *rheumatoid nodule* and a *gouty tophus* on physical examination?

A2. You can't! Usually aspiration or biopsy is needed, unless the gouty tophus drains to the surface.

Q3. So you thought I was going to ask you to examine the patient for typical deformities in the hand of a person with rheumatoid arthritis. Well, please examine the *rheumatoid foot.*

A3.
- Pes planus – inward rotation of the medial malleolus
- Loss of anterior arch – wide front part of foot
- Hallux valgus – bending of the big toe towards the second toe
- Cock-up deformities of the toes – flexion of the IP joint of the toes
- Dropped metatarsal leads - subluxation of the metatarsal heads

Q4. What are the poor *prognostic factors* for RA?

A4.
- Systemic features: weight loss, extra-articular manifestations
- Insidious onset
- Rheumatoid nodules
- Presence of rheumatoid factor more than 1 in 512

Source: Baliga RR. *Saunders/Elsevier* 2007, page 339.

Q5. A patient with rheumatoid arthritis (RA) is found to have *splenomegaly*. What are the causes of splenomegaly in this patient which are related to the RA?

A5.
- Adult – Felty syndrome
- Child – Still's disease
- Amyloidosis
- Associated SLE
- Beucellosis

Q6. What is *palindromic rheumatoid arthritis*?

A6.
- Acute recurrent arthritis, usually affecting one joint, with symptom-free intervals of days to months between attacks

Source: Baliga RR. *Saunders/Elsevier* 2007, page 345.

**7. Osteoarthritis (OA)**

Q1. In the context of osteoarthritis (OA), how do you distinguish between *Heberden's and Bouchard's nodes.*

A1.
- Painless nodules – DIP, Heberden nodes (DIP, HeberDen)

  PIP, Bouchard nodes

Q2. OK. Now distinguish between Bouchard nodes, which usually occur in OA, and *Haygarth's nodes*, which usually occur in rheumatic disorders such as rheumatoid.

A2.
- Haygarth nodes are inflammatory and thus painful and tender, not painless and degenerative, as are Bouchard's nodes in OA
- These nodes affect
  - Occiput
  - Elbows
  - Middle & proximal PIP joints
  - Knees
  - Ankles

"The road leading to a goal does not separate you from the destination; it is essentially a part of it"

Charles DeLint

## 8. Osteomalacia

Q1. What are the radiological signs of *osteomalacia* (loss of mineral from bone, with normal protein matrix).

A1.
- o Milkman fracture (aka looser zone) – tongue of radiotranslucency extending from the surface into the bone
- o Usually seen upper end of femur or humerus, or lower end of tibia
- o Bending of bones
- o Later, features of osteoporosis
    - Cortex thinning sclerosis of cortex
    - Thinning (translucency) of bone
    - ↓ number of trabeculae
    - Sclerosis of remaining trabeculae
    - Axial bones affected more than peripheral bones

## 9. Paget disease

Q1. Paget disease usually causes sclerotic lesions, but the exception may be the skull. What are the *bony changes in the skull* in Paget disease?

A1.
- o Well circumscribed area of translucency (rarefraction) (aka osteoporosis circumscripta)
- o Platybasia-indentation of the soft skull by vertebral column (odontoid process of the axis > 5 mm above chamberlain's line [Chambalain's line is a straight line drawn backwards from the hard palate to 5 mm above the odontoid process)

## 10. Psoriasis

Q1. How does *sacroilitis of psoriatic arthritis* differ from ankylosing spondylitis?

A1. In psoriatic arthritis, the syndesmophytes are usually from the internal and anterior surfaces of the vertebral bodies, and not from the margins of the bodies as is usually the case in ankylosing spondylitis

Source Baliga RR. *Saunders/Elsevier* 2007, page 343.

## 11. Signs

Q1. In the context of the diabetic patient, what is the significance of the *prayer sign*?

A1.

- Prayer sign- unability to oppose the flexor surfaces of the PIPs
- Diabetic stiff hand syndrome
- Flexion contracture and limited flexion of PIP joints
- Positive prayer sign
- Waxy, thick skin over the fingers

Q2. In the context of diffuse swelling of a finger, what are the non-traumatic causes of a *sausage-shaped digit*.

A2.

- Psoriatic arthritis
- Sarcoidosis

Source: Mangione S. *Hanley & Belfus* 2000, page 462.

Q3. In the context of pain along the radial side of the wrist, what is *Finkelstein sign*?

A3.
- o Tenosynovitis of tendons of the thumb passing over the radius bone causes pain
- o The pain is reproduced by placing the thumb in the palm of the hand, and wrapping the fingers around the thumb.
- o The wrist is deviated to the ulnar side.

Q4. What is *Behcet syndrome*?

A4. Aphthous ulcers in mouth and genitals, associated with arthritis, uvertis and various neurological disorders

Source: Mangione S. *Hanley & Belfus* 2000, page 67.

Q5. When a person's fingers are exposed to the cold, they may become pale, then blue from the arterial vasospasm and ischemia, then with redness from reperfusion. This latter phase from a decline in the spasm and therefore ischemia may be associated with pain and paresthesia as well as the redness. In some persons (20%) no cause/ association may be found, and this progression of white-blue-red is called Reynaud disease (i.e., Reynaud phenomenon, with no known underlying disorder. However, the Raynaud phenomenon may preceed a number of conditions.

Perform a focused physical examination for the causes of *Raynaud phenomenon*.

- ➢ MSK
  - o Rheumatoid arthritis
  - o Scleroderma
  - o Systemic lupus erythematosis
  - o Mixed connective disease
  - o Dermatomyositis
  - o Polymyositis

| | |
|---|---|
| ➢ Hematological disorders | o Cryoglobulinemia<br>o Polycythemia<br>o Monoclonal gammopathy |
| ➢ Arterial | o Compression<br>- Thoracic outlet syndrome<br>- Carpal tunnel syndrome<br>o Artherosclerosis<br>o Vasculitis<br>o Prinznetal angina |
| ➢ Drugs and toxins | |
| ➢ Endocrine disorders | o Hypothyroidism<br>o Acromegaly<br>o Addison disease |
| ➢ Pulmonary disorders | o Idiopathic pulmonary hypertension |
| ➢ Neurological | o Reflex sympathetic dystrophy |
| ➢ Life style | o Occupational use of percussion or vibratory tools (e.g. a jack hammer) |

Q6. Fluid is palpated over the anterior surface of the joint. In this context, what is the *shoulder pad sign*, and what is its usual cause?

A6.

- The shoulder pad syndrome is bilateral shoulder effusions.
- The usual cause of bilateral shoulder effusions is amyloidosis.

Q7. What is *De Quervain disease*?

A7.
- Tenosynovitis involving abductor policis longus and extensor policies brevis
-
- Patient complains of weakness of grip and pain at the base of the thumb which is aggravated by certain movements of the wrist

Adapted from: Filate W, et al. *The Medical Society, Faculty of Medicine, University of Toronto 2005,* page 137.

"The secret of the care of the patient is in the caring for the patient."

Peabody FW. Doctor and patient. Harvard University

Press: Campridge, MA, 1928

## Neurology

### 1. Ataxia/ gait

Q1. What simple maneuver performed during the physical examination will help to distinguish *cerebellar ataxia* from *sensory ataxia*?

A1. Ataxia (clumsiness) due to cerebellar lesions persists when the eyes are closed, whereas sensory ataxia improves when the eyes are open

Q2. In the context of a gait disturbance, what do you understand by term '*astasia abasia*'?

A2.
- Seen in psychogenic disturbances in which the patient is unable to walk or cannot stand.
- The patient falls far to the side on walking but usually regains balance before hitting the ground.
- The legs may be thrown out wildly or the patient may kneel with each step.

Q3. What do you understand by the term '*marche a petits pas*'?

A3.
- A gait in which the movement is slow and the patie walks with very short, shuffling and irregular steps, with loss of associated movements.
- Seen in normal-pressure hydrocephalus.
- This gait bears some resemblance to that seen in Parkinson's disease.

Source: Baliga RR. *Saunders/Elsevier* 2007, Case 61, page 181.

Q4. What hematological abnormalities may be associated with *chorea*?

A4.
- o Polycythemia vera
- o Neuroacanthocytosis (chorea – acanthocystosis)

Q5. What is *Hemiballismus*?

A5.
- o Sudden onset of unilateral, involuntary, flinging movements of the proximal upper limbs
- o Cardiovascular disease (source of emboli)
  - Atrial fibrillation
  - Valvular heart disease
  - Severe left ventricular dysfunction, travelling to the ipsilateral subthalamic nucleus of lungs and causing an infarction
- o Unilateral, involuntary, flinging movement of the proximal upper limbs

Source: Baliga RR. *Saunders/Elsevier* 2007, page 218.

**2. Bladder**

Q1. Name three neurological conditions in which bladder disturbances are rare.

A1.
- o Motor neuron disease
- o Subacute combined degeneration
- o Peripheral neuritis
- o Extrapyramidal disease

## 3. Cerebellum

Q1. Name the three parts of the cerebellum, and perform a focused physical examination to distinguish which part is causing the *ataxia*.

A1.
- Paleocerebellum - Gait ataxia (inability to do tandem walking): anterior lobe
- Aerchicerebellum - Truncal ataxia (drunken gait, titubation): flocculonodular or posterior lobe
- Neocerebellum - Limb ataxia, especially upper limbs and hyponiA1. lateral lobes

Source: Baliga RR. *Saunders/Elsevier* 2007, page 145.

Q2. What is *Benedikt syndrome*?

A2.
- Cerebellar signs on the side opposite the third nerve palsy (which is produced by damage to the nucleus itself or to the nerve fascicle).
- Due to a midbrain vascular lesion causing damage to the red nucleus, interrupting the dentatorubrothalamic tract from the opposite cerebellum.

## 4. Cranial nerve (CN)

Q1. In the context of a *blow-out fracture* of the floor of the orbit, what are the defects in the cranial nerves (CN)?

A1.
- Inferior rectus muscle CN??
- Numbness on side of injury CN V

Q2. In the context of cranial nerves V and VI, what is *Gradenigo syndrome*?

A2. Gradenigo's syndrome is involvement of CN V and VI, with facial pain and sixth nerve palsy, such as may occur as a complication of otitis media and periostitis of the petrous

Q3. In the presence of increased intracranial pressure, which two nerves give *a false-localizing sign* of a lower motor neuron (LMN)?

A3. Cranial nerves III and VI

Q4. Which cranial nerve (CN) is most susceptible to a *transient increase in intracranial pressure*, such as might occur with a subarachnoid hemorrhage?

A4. CN VI

Q5. What are the causes of *pin-point pupils*?

A5. Pin-point pupils are caused by

- Opiates
- Positive hemorrhage

Q6. What is '*Fisher one and a half syndrome*'?

A6. Horizontal eye movement is absent, and the other eye is capable only of abduction ("one and a half movements are paralyzed").

- The vertical eye movements and the pupils are normal.
- The cause is a lesion in the pontine region involving the medial longitudinal fasciculus and the parapontine reticular formation on the same side.
- This results in failure of conjugate gaze to the same side, impairment of adduction of the eye, and nystagmus on abduction of the other eye.

Source: Baliga RR. *Saunders/Elsevier* 2007, page 222.

Q7. What are the structures in close proximity to the *CN VI nucleus and fascicles*?

A7.
- Facial and trigeminal nerves
- Corticospinal tract
- Median longitudinal fasciculus
- Parapontine reticular formation
- Temporal bone

Source: Baliga RR. *Saunders/Elsevier* 2007, page 151.

Q8. Why can the patient with central damage to CN VII *wrinkle their foreheads*?

A8. Both sides of the cortex supply the LMN innervation of the upper half of the face

Q9. What are the causes of *Bell palsy*?

A9.
- Idiopathic
- Infection
  - Epstein Barr Virus (infectious mononucleosis)
  - Guillain-Barre syndrome
- Infiltration
  - Tumor of cerebellopontine angle
- Metabolic
  - Diabetes

Q10. Why can the patient with Bell palsy not wrinkle their foreheads?

A10. Bell palsy is a peripheral mononeuropathy of CN VII.
- Their peripheral nerve damage causes paralysis of both UMN and LMN, so the motor function of both upper and lower portions of the face are affected.
- The eyelid of the affected side cannot be closed

Q11. What is the difference between *Bell palsy and Bell phenomenon*?

A11.
- Bell phenomenon is the normal upwards rotation

of the orbit which occurs when the ipsilateral orbicularis muscle contracts when the person closes their eye, i.e., the eyelid closes; because the eyelid closes, the physiological synkinesis of the upward movement involuntary of the eye with the voluntary closure of the eyelid is not normally seen.

Source: Mangione S. *Hanley & Belfus* 2000, page 410.

Q12. In the context of CN VII, what are the *Raeder paratrigeminal syndrome*, and the *superior orbital fissure syndrome*?

A12.
- o Raeder's paratrigeminal syndrome - Severe retro-orbital pain succeeded by ipsilateral miosis and ptosis
- o Superior orbital fissure syndrome – Boring retro-orbital pain and paresis or cranial nerves III, IV, V and VI

Q13. Perform a focused physical examination to distinguish between an *upper vs lower motor neuron* damage to cranial nerve (CN) VII (facial nerve).

A13. Oh boy!
- o UMN (cortical damage) weakness of lower facial muscle on the opposite side as the damage.
- o LMN (damage to CN > VII): inability to wrinkle the forehead, close the eye tightly, or smile on the same side as the damage.

Source: Mangione S. *Hanley & Belfus* 2000, pages 409 and 410.

Q14. What is the sensory component of the *facial nerve* (CN VII), and what does it supply?

A14.
- o The nervus intermedius of Wrisberg
- o Taste sensation from the anterio two thirds of

the tongue

- Probably, cutaneous impulse from the anterior wall of the external auditory canal.

Source: Baliga RR. *Saunders/Elsevier* 2007, page 159 and 160.

Q15. How do you *localize* the site of the facial nerve palsy?

A15.
- Involvement of the nuclei in pons – associated ipsilateral sixth nerve palsy.
- Cerebellopontine angle lesion – associated fifth and eight nerve involvement.
- Lesion in the bony canal – loss of taste (carried by the lingual nerve) and hyperacusis (due to involvement of the nerve to stapedius.

Q16. What *reflexes* involve the facial nerve?

A16.
- Corneal reflex
- Palmomental reflex
- Sucking reflex

Q17. What is the neuroanatomical basis for only the *tongue and lower face* being affected in UMN-associated hemiplegia?

A17.
- All cranial nerve are innervated bilaterally, except the lower half of the face and tongue; thus all muscles except tongue and lower face escape in UMN hemiplegia

Q18. What are the *eponymous syndromes* of the lower cranial nerves (CN)?

A18.
- CN IX, X and XI
  - Vernet's syndrome: paresis due to extension of tumour into

the jugular foramen.

- CN IX to XII
  - Collet-Sicard syndrome: fracture of the floor of the posterior cranial fossa.

- CN IX to XII
  - Villaret's syndrome: ipsilateral paralysis of the last four cranial nerves and cervical sympathetic.

- CN X , XI
  - Syndrome of Schmidt

- CN XI, XII
  - Syndrome of Hughlings Jackson

Q19. Why is the hypoclossal nerve not part of the jugular foramen syndrome?

A19. CN XII leaves through the anterior condylar foramen.

Source: Baliga RR. *Saunders/Elsevier* 2007, pages 224 and 225.

Q20. Cranial nerve V (*trigeminal nerve*) is entirely sensory, except motor to which muscle?

A20. The masseter muscle for chewing

Q21. What is the *epomous syndrome* in which the third cranial nerve (CN III) is involved?

A21.
- o Weber syndrome: ipsilateral third nerve palsy with contralateral hemiplegia. The lesion is in the midbrain.
- o Benedikt syndrome: ipsilateral third nerve palsy with contralateral involuntary movement such as tremor, chorea and arthetos. It is due to a lesion of the red nucleus in the midbrain.
- o Claude syndrome: ipsilateral oculomotor paresis with contralateral ataxia and tremor. It is due to a lesion of the third nerve and red nucleus.
- o Nothnagel syndrome: unilateral oculomotor paralysis combined with ipsilateral cerebellar ataxia.

Source: Baliga RR. *Saunders/Elsevier* 2007, page 155.

**5. Coma**

Q1. What is the differential diagnosis of *coma* (Note: NOT the differential diagnosis of the causes of coma)?

A1.
- ➢ Locked-in-state
  - o Damage to junction between upper one third and lower two thirds of pons
  - o No function below the pons, but there may be enough RAS function for person to be awake
  - o Control of only CN III/VI (blinking eyes)
- ➢ Hysteric coma
  - o Hand dropping test, following gently to side
- ➢ Catatonic coma
  - o Preexisting depression, in which an intercurrent major illness then leads to catatonia

Source: Mangione S. *Hanley & Belfus* 2000, page 428.

### 6. Crossed hemiplegia

Q1. In the context of a crossed hemiplegia, what are the *Weber, Millard and Foville syndromes*?

A1.
- Weber's syndrome: ipsilateral lower motor neuron lesion of the oculomotor nerve with contralateral hemiplegia.
- Millard Gubler syndrome: lower motor neuron lesion of the abducens nerve which supplies the lateral rectus and contralateral hemiplegia.
- Foville's syndrome: in which there is a hemiplegia with paralysis of conjugate deviation towards the side of the lesion, i.e. the eyes are fixed towards the weak side; in a hemiplegia due to a lesion in the internal capsule, the eyes tend to be fixed away from the weak side.
- Hemiplegia on one side with weakness of muscles supplied by the lower cranial nerves (IX-XII) on the opposite side.

Source: Davey P. *Wiley-Blackwell* 2006, page 246.

### 7. CVA

Q1. From the physical examination, how would you be able to differentiate between an obstruction of *Heubner (medial striate) artery*, and a more distal occlusion of the anterior cerebral artery?

A1.
- Obstruction of Heubner artery (anterior damage to the limb of internal capsule and extrapyramidal nuclei)
  - Contralateral weakness and spasticity in the upper body
- Obstruction of ACA
  - Contralateral flaccid weakness of the leg

Q2. Why are the upper portions of the body affected less than the lower body by a vascular lesion of the *middle cerebral artery* (which supplies the internal capsule)?

A2. The fibers which supply the lower portion of the body are in the posterior portion of the internal capsule, and are supplied by only one vessel, whereas the fibers which supply the upper portion of the body are in the anterior portion of the internal capsule, which has a dual blood supply.

**8. Deep pain**

Q1. Do you wish to be really mean? What are the methods of *eliciting deep pain*?

A1.
- Abadie sign – the loss of pain sense in the Achilles tendon.
- Biernacki sign – the absence of pain on pressure on the ulnar nerve.
- Royal College Sign – too many questions on neurology.
- Pitres' sign – loss of pain on pressure on the testes.
- Haenel sign – analgesia to pressure on the eyeballs.

Source: Baliga RR. *Saunders/Elsevier* 2007, page 201.

**9. Deep tendon reflexes**

Q1. What is the location of a lesion which causes *hyporeflexia but no wasting*?

A1. A peripheral nerve lesion.

Q2. What are the causes of *absent knee and ankle jerks*, with an *extensor plantar response*?

A2..
- Sub-acute combined degeneration
- Syphilitic tabo-paresis
- Friedreich's ataxia
- Motor neurone disease

Source: Burton JL. *Churchill Livingstone* 1971, page 88.

Q3. What conditions demonstrate an up - *going plantar reflex* but *absent knee reflexes*?

A3.
- Friedreich's ataxia
- Multiple sclerosis
- Peripheral neuropathy in a stroke patient.
- Motor neuron disease.
- Conus medullaris-cauda equina lesion.
- Tabes dorsalis
- Subacute combined degeneration of the spinal cord

Q4. What is the mechanism?

A4. A mixture of cerebellar, pyramidal and dorsal column signs with a combination of pyramidal weakness with peripheral neuropathy.

Source: Baliga RR. *Saunders/Elsevier* 2007, pages 191 and 192.

Q5. Describe the abnormal reflexes which occur in Parkinsonism!

A5. That was a nasty trick: the deep tendon reflexes are normal

## 10. Delirium

Q1. In delirium, there is abnormal perception and motor activity. What is the difference between *hallucination and illusion*?

A1.
- Hallucination – sensory impression, without sensory stimulus
- Illusion – sensory impression which is incorrectly interpreted

## 11. Ear

Q1. What structural damage causes *Nystagmus*?

A1. Nystagmus is the involuntary oscillation of the eye. It is caused by damage to the mechanisms in the brain or brainstem for the coordination of eye movements (not due to damage to CN III, IV, VI).

Q2. Nystagmus may be horizontal, vertical or rotatory, and has a quick and slow component. The rhythmic movement of the extraocular muscles may arise from disease of the cerebellum, vestibularis or oculomslor system. And so, the question: how would you determine if *nystagmus* is "*physiological*"?

A2. Test for "optokinetic" nystagmus by having the person look at a rapidly rotating vertically striped drum.

## 12. Eye

Q1. In the context of blindness, what is *amaurosis fugax*?

A1.
- A transient monocular blindness due to episodic retinal ischemia, usually associated with ipsilateral carotid artery stenosis or embolism of the retinal arteries resulting in a sudden, and frequently complete, loss of vision in one eye.

Source: Jugovic PJ, et al. *Saunders/ Elsevier* 2004, page 150.

Q2. Why does *obstruction of the PCA* distal to the thalamic branch not affect the macula?

A2. Because the macula is supplied by both the MCA and the PCA

Q3. From the physical examination, how would you determine if the patient had *cortical blindness* (CB) from occlusion of the PCAs, versus damage to the optic tracts (OT), optic nerve (ON) or the retina (R)?

A3.

| Finding | OT/ON/R | CD |
|---|---|---|
| o Pupillary reflexes | + | normal |
| o Fundus | + | normal |
| o Awareness when light shone in eyes | + | no |

Q4. In the context of an abnormal examination of the eyes, what is *Eales' Disease*.

A4.
- Periodic vitreous hemorrhage and pre-retinal (subhyaloid) hemorrhages.
- Disease of young man attributed to tuberculosis periphlebitis.

Q5. What is the Argyll Robertson pupil; give its clinical features, explain the underlying neuroanatomy and provide a systemic approach to its causes.

A5.

- Definition: The Argyll Robertson pupil is a pupil which reacts to accommodation, but not to light
- Neuroanatomy
  - Unlike the pupillary light reflex, the efferent fibers of the accommodation reflex do not pass through the ciliary ganglion
  - Thus, a lesion of the oculomotor (CN III) nerve fibers damages the area of the ciliary ganglion will prevent the light reflex but not the accommodation reflex
  - Sympathetic innervation may also be impaired
- Clinical features
  - Pupils react to accommodation but not to light
  - Pupils are not always small
  - Pupils may react a little to light (constriction), but with constriction not being maintained
  - Small irregular pupil
  - Patchy atrophy of iris
  - Depigmentation of iris
- Causes
  - Damage to the midbrain, including
  - Infection
    - Syphilis (GPI, or tabes dorsalis)
    - Diabetes
    - Tumor
    - Vascular lesion
    - Postencephalitic parkinsonism
    - Polyneuritis

Q6. What is the *Holmes-Adie pupil?*

A6.
- o Large pupil
- o Reacts only slowly to accommodation, but not to light
- o Unilateral
- o Usually occurs in women
- o Associated with slow deep tendon reflexes

Q7. Be prepared to *differentiate* between the pupils in Argyll Robertson versus Holmes-Adie syndrome.

A7. Please see answers above

Q8. How may you distinguish clinically between CN III palsy and exophthalmos due to a cavernous sinus thrombosis or aneurysm versus a tumor of the orbit?

A8.
- o With a tumor of the orbit
  - The CN III palsy and exophthalmos are usually bilateral
  - Associated chemosis (red, edematous conjunctive)
  - Associated papilledema

Q9. In what eye disease is it not possible to properly assess anisocoria?

A9. With iritis, the patient may have so much photophobia that it is not possible to determine if the size of the pupils is not equal.

Q10. In the context of the Argyll Robertson pupil (ARP), what is Adie pupil (AP)?

A10.

| | Light | Accommodation |
|---|---|---|
| ARP | No | Yes |
| AP | No | No |

Q11. Give the translational neuroanatomical basis for the Marcus Gunn pupil (afferent pupillary defect).

A11.
- Afferent stimulus from
  - Disease eye weak
  - Contralateral healthy eye strong

- Efferent system
  - Normal in diseased and healthy eye

- With the swinging flashlight test
  - Light in normal eye
    - Normal pupil constricts
  - Light taken away from normal eye to diseased eye
    - Loss of constriction signal from to normal eye
    - No afferent pathway from diseased eye to cause constriction of pupil on that side
    - The pupil in the affected eye initially dilates in response to light, rather than constricting as would be normal

Q12. In the context of the pupil of the eye, distinguish between "near-light dissociation" (NLD) and "light-near dissociation" (LNA)

A12.

| Pupil reaction to | NLD | LND |
|---|---|---|
| ➢ Light | Yes | No |
| ➢ Synkinesis | No | Yes |

Adapted from: McGee SR. *Saunders/Elsevier* 2007, page 216.

Q13. In Horner syndrome, how would you differentiate clinically whether the lesion is above the superior ganglion (peripheral) or below the superior cervical ganglion (central)?

A13.

| Test | Above | Below |
|---|---|---|
| Sweating | Such lesions may not affect sweating at all as the main outflow to the facial blood vessels is below the superior cervical ganglion | Such lesion affect sweating over the entire head, neck, arm, and upper trunk Lesions in the lower neck affect sweating over the entire face |

Source: Baliga RR. *Saunders/Elsevier* 2007, page 127.

Q14. How would you distinguish congenital from non-congenital Horner syndrome?

A14. Incongenital Horner's, there are all the usual features of miosis, ptosis, enopthalmos, and elevation of the lower lip, plus there would be heterochromia of the iris (i.e. the iris remains grey-blue).

Q15. In the patient with ipsilateral Horner syndrome and contralateral loss of pain and temperature sensation, what is Wollenberg syndrome?

A15. Wollenberg syndrome is also known as the lateral medullary syndrome, which usually presents with the above features in the person who has suffered a stroke.

Q16. Distinguish between Argyll Robertson pupils (ARP), and the pupils of the patients with aberrant regeneration of CN III (AR III).

A16.

| Clinical | AR III | ARP |
|---|---|---|
| o Constriction of pupil during convergence, but not to light | Unilateral | Bilateral |
| o Associated anisocoria, ptosis, diplopia | Yes | No |

Q17. What is the 'reversed' Argyll Robertson pupil?

A17.
- o The pupil react to light but not to accommodation
- o Seen in parkinsonism caused by encephalitis lethargic

Q18. What causes *miosis*?

A18.
- o Old age
- o Pilocarpine (treatment for glaucoma)

Q19. What non-neurological conditions cause an *eccentric pupil?*

A19.
- Trauma
- Iritis

Q20. Unequal size of the pupil (anisocoria) may occur congenitally. In the comatose patient, how do you determine by physical examination if the anisocorm is due to a pathological process?

A20. Pathological anisocoria is asymmetry of the pupils plus loss of reaction of the pupils to light

Q21. What are causes of *red eye*?

A21.

- Conjunctiva
  - Conjunctivitis
  - Allergic
  - Viral
  - Bacterial
- Cornea
  - Inflammation of the cornea or keratits
- Episclera
  - Episcleritis is inflammation of the connective tissue between the sclera and conjunctiva
- Sclera
  - Inflammation of the sclera (scleritis)
  - Indicates an underlying systemic disease; such as connective tissue disease

| | |
|---|---|
| ➢ Iris and ciliary body | ○ Acute iridocyclitis is inflammation of both the iris and ciliary body |
| ➢ Adnexal structures | ○ Tear or sebaceous glands; both dacryocystitis and styes are common disorders |
| ➢ Intraocular | ○ Acute glaucoma |

Source: Mangione S. Hanley & Belfus 2000, page 103.

Q22. What is the significance of loss of pulsation of the retinal arteries?

A22. None. In the retina, the veins (not the arteries) show pulsations. Loss of retinal vein pulsations suggests an increased intraocular pressure (papilledema).

Q23. When are the *sclera blue*?

A23.
- In newborns
- Pseudo-pseudohypoparathyroidism
- Marfan's syndrome
- Osteogenesis imperfecta (hallmark)
- Anemia (especially iron deficiency)

Source: Mangione S. *Hanley & Belfus* 2000, page 83.

Q24. When is the red eye *conjunctivitis and not uveitis*?

A24
- Conjunctivitis
  - Diffuse red edemators, sclera and palpebral conjunctivae
  - Discharge (bacterial-purulent/mucopurulent; viral and chemical – watery discharge
  - Discomfort, with scratchy feeling of sand in eye
- Uveitis
  - Circumcorneal injected vessels (at the limbus) (aka ciliary flush)
  - Photophobia
  - Deep, aching pain, not relieved with a topical anesthetic

Source: Mangione S. *Hanley & Belfus* 2000, page 83.

Q25. What is *Horner syndrome*?

A25. Horner syndrome

- Signs
- Miosis
- Ptosis (at rest, but not on looking upwards)
- Anhydrosis
- Lack of tears
- Causes
  - Cervical lymphadenopathy
  - Lesions of medulla
    - Syringomyelia
    - Syringobulbia
    - Vascular lesions

Q26. In the context of Horner syndrome, and using only physical examination of the eye, distinguish between *congenital versus acquired* causes.

A26. Heterochromia (different pigmentation in the ireses of the eyes) is common in congenital Horner's, but rare in acquired disease.

Source: Mangione S. *Hanley & Belfus* 2000, page 85.

Q27. Give four conditions which may cause *spasms of conjugate deviation of the eye*.

A27.

- At the beginning of a seizure
- At the beginning of CVA
  - Early, head and eye turn away from the side of the lesion
  - Later, head and eye turn towards the side of the lesion
- Oculogyric crisis in encephalitis lethargica
- Hysteria

Q28. What three muscle groups are supplied by the oculomotor nerve (CN III)?

A28.

- All eye muscles, except lateral rectus (LR) and superior oblique (SO)
- Eye is rotated out by LR and down by SO
- Levator palpebrae superioris
- Constrictor muscle of pupils
- Loss of constrictor muscle leads to unopposed sympathetic effects on pupil

Q29. The cranial nerves to the muscles of the eye run closely together, so then two or three may be affected by the same lesion. What is the lesion which damages CN IV, and usually not CN III and VI?

A29. Aneurysm of PCA

Q30. What is the difference between hyphema and hypopyon?

A30. Hyphema is blood, and hypopyon is pus in the anterior chamber of the eye

Q31. What are the neurological conditions causing ptosis?

A31.

- CN III palsy
- Horner's syndrome
- Myasthenia gravis

Source: Mangione S. *Hanley & Belfus* 2000,

Q32. Of course, we all know that blue slerae are usually associated with ostegenesis imperfecta. But name other associations.

A32.

- Anemia
- Marfan's syndrome
- Pseudo-pseudo hypoparathyroidism
- Newborns, small children, some "normal" adults

Q33. A “fixed pupil” is a pupil which does not react to light or to accommodation. A fixed pupil which is dilated may be due to iritis or to oculomotor (CN III) lesion. How can you distinguish between the two by examining the eyes?

A33.
- Iritis
  - Fixed, dilated, irregular pupil
  - Does not react to light or accommodation
- Retrobulbar neuritis
  - Fixed dilated pupil
  - Reacts slowly to direct light

Q34. You are familiar with how to examine CN III. Perform an examination for "aberrant regeneration" of CN III.

A34. Pathogenesis: After damage to the third nerve (from trauma, aneurysms, or tumors but not ischemia), regenerating fibers originally destined for the medial rectus muscle may instead reinnervate the pupillary constrictor

- Clinical
  - Unilateral pupillary constriction during convergence but no reaction to light. Unlike Argyll Robertson pupils, however, this finding is unilateral
  - Anisocoria, ptosis, and diplipia

Q35. Give one cause of intermittent Horner syndrome.

A35. Easy- Migraine.

Q36. Give three examples of physical findings of the *optic disc*, and their interpretation.

A36. Normally the disc is pales, sharply defined but with slight blurring of nasal margin, and slightly paler on temporal than on the nasal side

- Increased temporal palor
  - Multiple sclerosis
- Increased nasal blurring
  - Papilledema
- Pink disc
  - Papilledema
  - Papillitis
- Pale disk
  - Optic atrophy

Q37. Give four causes of *retinal artery microaneurysms.*

A37.
- Diabetes
- Systemic hypertension
- Thrombosis of retinal vein
- Sickle cell anemia

Q38. Is the *cornea reflex* lost if a patient has weakness of the face as a result of damage to the facial nerve and LMV lesion?

A38. No, since there is bilateral innervation of the orbicularis oculi

Q39. What is the neuroanatomy which explains the corneal reflex?

A39.
- The sensory fibers of the CN V (touch, proprioception) enter the brainstem and cross the midline to ascent in the medial lemniscus to the thalamus and cerebral cortex

Sensory nuclei in pons CN V → brainstem → decussate → medial lemniscus → thalamus and cerebral cortex
Sensory and motor V → leave the pons V cross the cerebellopontine angle → sensory root in a large ganglion at the apex of the petrous temporal bone → sensory V accompanies CN III, IV, and VI in the cavernous sinus

Q40. From the physical examination of the eye, how can you distinguish between *retrobulbar neuritis, and papilledema*?

A40.
- Retrobulbar neuritis
  - Early severe reduction in vision
  - Central scotoma affecting
  - Blind spot
  - Slow direct light reaction
  - Papilledema with papillitis
  - Macula (fixation spot)
  - Rapid reaction to consensual light
  - Normal accommodation

- Papilledema
  - Late, milder loss of vision
  - Larger blind spot
  - Increased nasal blurring
  - Pink disc
  - Secondary optic atrophy
  - Smaller peripheral field of vision
  - Macula (fixation spots) is unaffected
  - If papilledema is severe, there may be hemorrhage and exudates

Q41. From the examination of the ocular blood vessels at fundoscopy, how can you *distinguish an artery from a vein*?

A41.
- As compared to vein, the artery is
  - Slightly tortous
  - Smaller (2.3)
  - Lighter in the centre than at the periphery
  - May have disease associated changes, e.g. silver wiring, hemorrhages

Q42. From fundoscopic examination of the ocular vessels, how can you distinguish between *choriodosis* and *retinitis*?

A42. Choroidosis – exudate is under the vessel (superficial to the exudate)
Retinitis – exudate interrupts the vessel

**13.Foramen magnum**

Q1. The signs of *foremen magnum* pressure cone caused by increased pressure in the foramen magnum may be micked by what bony conditions?

A1.
- Invagination of the base of the stull into the upper cervical spine, from
  - Congenital anomaly
  - Osteomalacia
  - Paget's disease
- Fusion of the cervical vertebrae
  - Congenital anomaly (aka Klippel-Feil deformity)

Q2. Many conditions may increase intracranial pressure (e.g. hemorrhagic stroke, brain abscess or tumor with cerebral), and cause "coning" ( nastral-candal herniation of the uncus of the temporal lobe, followed by compression of the brainstem). Your question: trace the signs which display the layer-by-layer loss of function which occur with the progression of *coning*.

A2.
- Ipsilateral cerebral posturing
  - Decortication, then
  - Decerebration
- Loss of painful stimuli
- Ipsilateral dilated pupil
- Ipsilateral loss of oculo cephalic reflex ("doll's head")
- Corneal reflex tests become positive
- Contralateral paratonic muscle resistance, and positive contralateral plantar extensor ("Babinski") reflex.

Source: Mangione S. *Hanley & Belfus* 2000, page 429.

**14.Frontal lobe**

Q1. In the context of the frontal lobe of the cerebral cortex, what is the *Foster Kennedy syndrome*?

A1. Optic atrophy on the side of compression of the optic nerve by the frontal lobe, and papilledema of the opposite eye resulting from increased intracranial pressure.

Q2. What is the physical sign which is considered to be pathognomonic of a *tumor of the frontal lobe*?

A2. The “grasp” reflex

Q3. What are the physical findings found in a person with *Pick presenile dementia*?

A3. That’s right: Good answer – Same findings as disturbed function of the frontal lobe of the cerebral cortex

**15.Headache**

Q1. Give the *serious causes of headache* in which neuroimaging findings may be normal.

A1.
- Giant cell or temporal arteritis
- Glaucoma
- Trigeminal or glossopharyngeal neuralgia
- Lesions around sella turcica
- Sentinel bleed of aneurysm (warning leak)
- Inflammation, infection, or neoplastic invasion of leptomeninges
- Cervical spondylosis
- Pseudotumor cerebri
- Low intracranial pressure syndromes

Source: Ghosh AK. *Mayo Clinic Scientific Press* 2008, Table 19-10, page 759.

**16.LMN**

Q1. You suspect that your patient has a disorder of the motor system of the upper limbs. What is the use of tapping the brachioradialis and biceps muscles to accentuate the finding of *fasciculations*?

A1. None! Fasciculations are spontaneous; movements from a local stimulus is not spontaneous. Even if movement occurs, the movement may have nothing to do with fasciculations.

Source: Talley NJ, et al. *Maclennan & Petty Pty Limited* 2003, page 391.

**17.Medulla**

Q1. Where is the lesion in the *lateral medullary syndrome*?

A1.
- Infarction of a wedge-shaped area of the lateral aspect of the medulla and inferior surface of the cerebellum
- The deficits are caused by involvement of one side of the nucleus ambiguous, trigeminal nucleus, vestibular nuclei, cerebellar peduncle, spinothalamic tract and autonomic fibers.

Q2. Which *vessels* may be occluded?

A2. Any of the following five vessels
- Posterior inferior cerebellar artery
- Vertebral artery
- Superior, middle or inferior lateral medullary arteries

Q3. Why does a lesion of the lateral side of the medulla cause ipsilateral loss of sensation of the face, but contralateral loss of sensation (pain and temperature)?

A3. A lesion of the lateral side of the medulla affects the descending tract of cranial nerve V (trigeminal nerve) before it crosses in the cranial portion of the spinal cord, whereas the fibers of the lateral spinothalamic tract cross after they enter the spinal cord.

Q4. What is the *medial medullary syndrome*?

A4.
- Occlusion of the lower basilar artery of vertebral arter
- Ipsilateral lesions result in paralysis and wasting o the tongue.
- Contralateral lesions result in hemiplegia and loss of vibration and joint position sense.

Source : Baliga RR. *Saunders/Elsevier* 2007, page 230.

## 18. Meninges

Q1. What are the typical neurological lesions associated with *leptomeningeal lesions*?

A1.
- Cerebral
  - Headache
  - Seizures
  - Focal neurologic signs
- Cranial nerve
- Any cranial nerve can be affected, especially CN III, IV, VI, and VII
- CN VII is often affected in Lynne disease
- Radicular (radiculoneuropathy or radiculomyelopathy) - neck and back pain as well as radicular pain and spinal cord signs

Source: Ghosh AK. *Mayo Clinic Scientific Press* 2008, page 762.

## 19. Meningismus

Q1. We all know that meningitis will cause meningismus, symptoms of headache, photophobia and nuchal rigidity. But what other non-musculoskeletal (i.e. neurological ) conditions may cause a *stiff neck*?

A1.
- Intracerebral bleed
- Posterior fossa tumor

## 20. Multiple sclerosis (MS)

Q1. What are the prognostic markers that predict more *severe multiple sclerosis*?

A1.
- Progressive disease from the onset of symptoms.
- Frequent relapses in the first two years.
- Motor and cerebellar signs at presentation to neurologist.
- Short interval between the first two relapses.
- Male gender.
- Poor recovery from relapse.
- Multiple cranial lesions on T2-weighted MRI at presentation.

Source : Baliga RR. *Saunders/Elsevier* 2007, page 178.

Q2. Give there examples of neurologist conditions which undergo *remission and relapses*.

A2.
- Multiple sclerosis
- Infections (of CNS)
- Myasthenia gravis

**21. Myasthenia gravis**

Q1. What is *myasthenic crisis*?

A1. Exacerbation of MG, especially bulbar and respiratory involvement, leading to need for ventilation.

Q2. What is *cholinergic crisis*?

A2. Excessive sensitivity to cholinergics in MG, such as in myasthenic crisis, with excessive salivation, confusion, lacrimation, miosis, pallor and collapse.

**22. Myopathy**

Q1. What conditions cause both a *proximal myopathy* and a *peripheral neuropathy*?

A1.

- Paraneoplastic syndrome
- Alcohol
- Hypothyroidism
- Connective tissue diseas

Source: Talley NJ, et al. *Maclennan & Petty Pty Limited* 2003, Tables 10.29 and 10.30, page 428.

**23. Nerve roots**

Q1. Which deep tendon reflexes are affected in *L5 lesions*?

A1. The knee jerk is innervated through nerve root L3 and L4, so this reflex remains normal with a L5 disc protrusion

Q2. Why does protrusion of *L4-L5 or L5-S1* never cause UMN signs?

A2. The spinal cord ends at L2, and below L2 is the Cauda equina consists of all the nerve roots below L2, L4-L5 or L5-S1 prolapse cannot cause UMN signs.

Q3. Distinguish ulnar lesions from T1 root lesions (*abductor pollicis brevis*).

A3. The thumb is moved vertically against resistance, with the hand supine.

Q4. In the context of cervical radiculopathy. What is the "*Spurling test*" or "*neck compression test*"?

A4. In this test, the clinician turns and tilts the patient's head and neck toward the painful side and then adds a compressive force to the top of the head. Aggravation of pain is a positive response!

Source: McGee SR. *Saunders/Elsevier* 2007, page 776.

Q5. What is the area of the skin (*dermatome*) which is supplied by the following nerve fibers originating from a single dorsal nerve root:

A5. $C_6$ - Thumb | $L_5$ - Top of foot

$T_4$ - Nipple lime | $S_1$ - Bottom of foot

$T_{10}$ - Umbilicus | $S_{2-4}$ - Perineum

Source: Mangione S. *Hanley & Belfus* 2000, page 414.

Q6. From the history, how do you distinguish *radiculopathy for peripheral neuropathy*?

A6.
- o Peripheral neuropathy - changes in motor and sensory function (denervation causing LMN lesion with weakness, atrophy, fasciculations)
- o Radiculopathy - motor and sensory loss, plus pain

Q7. What are the causes of *a claw hand* (all fingers clawed)?

A7.
- o Ulnar and median nerve lesion (ulnar nerve palsy alone causes a claw-like hand)
- o Brachial plexus lesion (C8-T1)
- o Other neurological disease – e.g. syringomyelia, polio
- o Ischemic contracture (late and severe)
- o Rheumatoid arthritis (advanced, untreated disease)

Source: Talley NJ, et al. *Maclennan & Petty Pty Limited* 2003, Table 10.13, page 403; Baliga RR. *Saunders/Elsevier* 2007, page 209.

Q8. What are the clinical tests of the function of the RAS (*reticular activating system*)?

A8.
- ➢ Oculocephalic reflex ("doll's eye" reflex)
- ➢ Ostimulation of receptors in middle ear, afferent signals in CN VIII to brainstem at the cerebellar - pontine angle; efferent pathway to CN III/VI (upper pons), with III and VI connected by MLF (midbrain)
- ➢ (medial longitudinal fasciculons), which is surrounded by RAS
    - o thus, damage to RAS affects MLF, which in turn leads to loss of RAS function in the pons, indicating brainstem damage

- Corneal reflex
    - painful sensory input from CN V, which enters brainstem in pons and medulla; CN VII is the efferent pathway to the orbicularis muscle, causing blinking of the eye

Adapted from: Mangione S. *Hanley & Belfus* 2000, page 425.

**24.Neurofibromatosis**

Q1. In the person with neurofibromatosis, what is a *Lisch nodule*?

A1. Lisch nodules are melanocytic hamartomas, well-defined, dome-shaped elevations projecting from the surface of the iris and are clear to yellow and brown.

**25.Parietal lobe**

Q1. In the context of the parietal lobe, what is *Gerstmann syndrome*?

A1.
- Confusion of the right and left side of the body
- Lack of ability to identify the figures
- Acalculia

**26.Parkinsonism**

Q1. How do you distinguish clinically from *rigidity and spasticity*?

A1.
- Rigidity
    - Increased muscle tone through all parts of the movement of the joint
    - Usually seen in degenerative neurological conditions e.g. Parkinsonism
- Spasticity

- Increasing muscle tone as muscle is stretched more and more, followed by a giveaway phenomenon of protection relaxation, leading to a jack-knife loss of tone
- Usually due to damage to the pyramidal (corticspinal) tract

Adapted from: Mangione S. *Hanley & Belfus* 2000, page 414.

Q2. In the content of mild Parkinsonism, what other neurological or endocrine conditions may give a slightly *abnormal facies*?

A2.
- Neurological
  - Mild pseudobulbar palsy
- Endocrine
  - Hypothyroidism
  - Acromegaly
  - Paget's disease

Source: Davies IJT. *Lloyd-Luke (medical books) LTD* 1972, page 290.

Q3. What is the difference between *rigidity, spascity, gegenhalten, tardive dyskinesia and the wheelchair sign*?

A3.
- Rigidity indicates increased tone affecting opposing muscle groups equally, and is present throughout the range of passive movement. When smooth it is called 'leadpipe' rigidity, and when intermittent in termed 'cog-wheel' rigidity. It is common in extrapyrimidal syndromes. Wilson's disease and Creutzfeld-Jakab disease.
- Spasticity of the clasp-knife type is characterized by increased tone which is maximal at the beginning of movement and suddenly decreases as passive movement is continued. It occurs chiefly in floors of the upper limb and etensors of

the lower limb (antigravity muscle).

- Gehenhalten, or paratonia, is where the increased muscle tone varies and becomes worse the more the patient tries to be relaxed.
- Tardive dyskinesia is seen in patients taking neuroleptics. Its manifestations are orofacial dyskinesia such as smacking, chewing lip movements, discrete dystonia or choreiform movements and, rarely, rocking movements.
- Withdrawal of the "Wheelchair sign" in Parkinson's - patients with advanced disease and "on-off" motor fluctuations require a wheelchair when "off" and when "on" are seen to walk about (sometimes pushing the chair!). These patients are rarely permanently wheelchair-bound; in contrast, those who never leave their wheelchair usually do not have Parkinson's disease.

Adapted from: Baliga RR. *Saunders/Elsevier* 2007, page 139 and McGee SR. *Saunders/Elsevier* 2007, pages 139 and 140.

Q4. Some persons with Parkinson disease have other neurological deficits. These are called "*Parkinson plus syndromes*", Give 4 examples.

A4.
- Steele – Richardson – Olszewski disease (akinesia, aial rigidity of the neck, bradyphrenia, supranuclear palsy)
- Multiple system atrophy (MSA)
  - Olivopontocerebellar degeneration
  - Strionigral degeneration
  - Progressive autonomic failure (Shy – Drager syndrome)
- Basal ganglia calcification
- Give up and switch to something else

Source: Baliga RR. *Saunders/Elsevier* 2007, page 142.

## 27. Peripheral nerves

Q1. What is the difference between *neuropraxia, axonotmesis, and neurotmesis*?

A1. I don't really care. (Not a good response!)

- Neurapraxia - concussion of the nerve after which a complete recovery occurs.
- Axonotmesis the axon is severed, but the myelin sheath is intact and recovery may occur.
- Neurotmesis - the nerve is completely severed, and the prognosis for recovery is poor.

Source: Baliga RR. *Saunders/Elsevier* 2007, page 211.

Q2. Distinguish between *median and ulnar nerve defects* affecting the hands:

A2. The Median nerve supplies

- Motor (mnemonic LOAF)
  - Lateral two lumbricals
  - Opponens pollicis
  - Abductor pollicis brevis
  - Flexor pollicis brevis
- Sensory to the radial 3½ digits
- Ulnar nerve supplies all the rest

Source: Burton JL. *Churchill Livingstone* 1971, page 84.

Q3. In the patient with symptoms and signs suggestive of peripheral neuropathy, what is the important symptom which suggests that the disease is at the *nerve root*?

A3. Pain! Severe pain which may radiate down the arms or legs

Source: Mangione S. *Hanley & Belfus* 2000,

## 28. Posterior root ganglion

Q1. What are the commonest causes of posterior root ganglial conditions:

A1.
- Diabetes
- Tabes dorsalis
- Carcinomatous neuropathy

## 29. Speech

Q1. What are the differences between *receptive and expressive aphasia*?

A1. Aphasia is an acquired disturbance of language

| | |
|---|---|
| ➢ Receptive aphasia (sensory, fluent or Wernicke's aphasia) | ○ Lesion in temporal or parietal lobe<br>○ Jumbled words<br>○ Difficulty naming objects<br>○ Poor comprehension of spoken or written words |
| ➢ Expressive aphasia (motor, non-fluent or Brocca's aphasia) | ○ Lesion in frontal lobe<br>○ Good comprehension of spoken or written words<br>○ Slow, monosyllabic sentences |

Q2. What is dysarthria, and what are its causes?

A2. Dysarthria is the poor articulation of words

- Causes
  - Brain
    - Injury
  - Muscles of phonation
    - Paralysis

- Spasticity
  - Emotional stress

Q3. What *dysarthrias* may be of psychological origin?

A3. Stuttering and stammering

Q4. What is *cerebellar speech*?

A4. Slow irregular speech, with sudden changes in speed and volume

**30.Spinal cord**

Q1. In the context of spinal cord, what is *paraplegia-in-flexion*?

A1.
- Paraplesia-flexion is seen in partial transaction of the cord where the limbs are involuntarily flexed at the hips and knees because the extensors are more paralyzed than the flexors.
- In complete transaction of the spinal cord, the extrapyramidal tracts are also affected and hence no voluntary movement of the limb is possible, resulting in paraplegia-in-extension.

Source: Baliga RR. *Saunders/Elsevier* 2007, page 116.

Q2. In the context of a *prolapsed intervertebral disc*, what nerve roots supply the pain which radiates to

- Lateral side of lower leg, and medial side of the foot
- Lateral side of the foot, and sole of the foot

A2. No, not L5 and S1!

- Pain from a prolapsed intervertebral disc does not radiate in the cutaneous distribution of the nerve root

- However, numbness and/or tingling (paraesthesiae) may occur along the appropriate cutaneous distribution of L5/S1

Q3. What is the *triad of symptoms* which suggest spinal cord disease?

A3.
- Sensory level, a band of sensory change around the chest or abdomen
  - or a sharp level below which sensation is lost
- Distal
  - usually symmetric weakness
- Bowel and bladder changes

Source: Mangione S. *Hanley & Belfus* 2000, page 418.

**31.Spinocerebellar**

Q1. In addition to Friedreich ataxia, what are other syndromes with *spinocerebellar degeneration*?

A1.
- Roussy-Levy disease: hereditary spinocerebellar degeneration with atrophy of lower limb muscles and loss of deep tendon reflexes.
- Refsum's disease
- Machado-Joseph disease – dominant inheritance (first described in families of Portuguese origin)
  - Progressive ataxia, ophthalmoparesis, spasticity, dystonia, amyotrophy and parkinsonism.
- Dentatorubral pallidoluysian atrophy, similar to Machado-Joseph disease but maps on the short arm of chromosome 12 rather than 14.

Source: Baliga RR. *Saunders/Elsevier* 2007, page 193.

## 32. Syringomyelia

Q1. In patients with *syringomyelia* affecting the middle of the cervical cord, what is the neuroanatomical basis for the observation that the sensation of pain and temperature is lost from only the upper part of the face, and not also from the lower face?

A1.
- o The sensory fibers of the trigeminal nerve (CN V) which carry pain and temperature enter the brainstem and descend to the level of CN III (third cervical segment)
- o From C3, the V1 fibers cross the midline, and then ascend in the lateral spinothalamic tract (LST)
- o The lowest fibers in LST supply the upper part of the face

V1 → brainstem → descend to C3 → decussate → ascend in the LST

Q2. What is the difference between *hydromyelia* (aka syringobulbia) and syringomyelia?

A2.
- o Hydromyelia is the expansion of the ependyma-lined central canal of the spinal cord.
- o Syringomyelia is the formation of a cleft-like cavity in the inner portion of the cord. Both these lesions are associated with

Q3. What are the *clinical features* of syringobulbia?

A3.
- o Dissociated sensory loss of the face of the 'onion-skin' pattern (extending from behind forwards, converging on the nose and upper lip).
- o Vertigo (common symptom).
- o Wasting of the small muscles of the tongue (important physical sign).
- o The process may be limited to the medullary region.
- o The main cranial nerve nuclei involved are those of the

fifth, seventh, ninth and tenth cranial nerves.

**33. TIA/ CVA**

Q1. What is the difference between *TIA* and reversible ischemic neurological deficit (*RIND*)?

A.
- TIA is a stroke syndrome with neurological symptoms lasting from a few minutes to as long as 24 hours, followed by complete functional recovery.
- RIND is a condition in which a person has neurological abnormalities similar to acute completed stroke, but the deficit disappears after 14 to 36 hours, leaving few or no detectable neurological sequelae.

Source: Jugovic PJ, et al. *Saunders/ Elsevier* 2004, page 150.

**34. Uvula**

Q1. In the context of looking at the anatomy of the oropharynx, what abnormalities are you looking for in the *uvula*?

A1.
- Absence
    - Congenital
    - Surgical - UPPP (uvulopalatinopharyngoplasty) for obstructive sleep apnea
- Bifid
    - Occult cleft palate
    - Normal variant

Q2. In the context of examining the uvula, what is *Mueller sign.*

A2. Rhythmic pulsatile movement of uvula seen in chronic aortic regurgitation

Adapted from: Mangione S. *Hanley & Belfus* 2000, page 123.

Q3. When you ask the patient to say "Ahh", what structures are you looking at?

A3. See diagram

*Anatomy of the oropharynx*

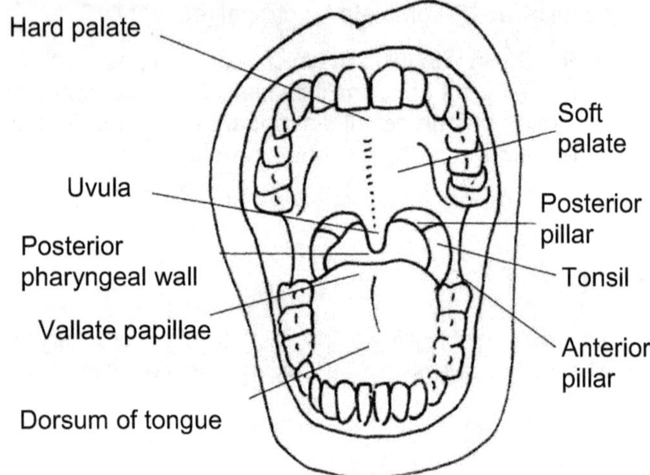


Source: Mangione S. *Hanley & Belfus* 2000, page 123.

**Miscellaneous**

Q1. You say that the patient "looks his/her *stated age*. But what conditions make you look older or younger that you actually are?

A2.
- Older
  - Smoking
  - Drinking in excess
  - Sunlight in excess
  - Chronic illness/cancer
  - Progeria (pathological acceleration of aging)
- Younger
  - Hypogonadism
  - Panhypopituitarism
  - You wish!

Adapted from: Mangione S. *Hanley & Belfus* 2000, page 11.

**1. HIV**

Q1. In the context of a person with HIV/AIDs, what is *eosinophilic folliculitis*?

A1. An infection of hair follicles, typically papular, pruritic and seen in HIV-infected persons

Q2. What is the nature of the interaction between HAV and HIV?

A2.
- ↑ HAV RNA titers
- Longer viremia
- ↑ AST / ALT
- Clinical outcome of HAV unchanged
- HAV vaccination is safe, but less immunogenic

Q3. What is the nature of the interation between HCV and HIV?

A3.
- o Prevalence of HCV in HIV is common drug users, hemophiliacs, about ¾ non-drug users, MSM, about 1/20
- o ↑ HCV RNA
- o ↑ ALT / AST
- o ↑ risk of cirrhosis
- o ↑ HCC

HCV does not cause progression of HIV disease

Q4. Give 4 risk factors for the clinical worsening of HCV in HIV.

A4.
- o ↑ age at infection
- o ↑ ALT
- o ↑ inflammatory activity
- o ↑ alcohol (>50 g/day)
- o ↓ CD (< 500 cell/mm)
- o Steatohepatitis

Q5. About 90% of AIDS patients are infected with HBV. What is the nature of the relationship between *HIV and HBV*?

A5.
- ➢ HBsAg
  - o Reapprearance of previously cleared HBsAg
  - o Reinfection or reactivation of HBV
  - o Chronic carrier state has less HBV-related liver injury, and only mild changes in serum hepatic biochemistry and liver histology
- ➢ HBeAg
  - o ↑ expression of HBeAg
  - o ↑ DNA polymerase
  - o ↑ HBeAg
- ➢ Carrier
  - o ↑ prevalence of highly infectious chronic carrier state

- ➢ Acute HBV flares
  - o Fulminant hepatic failure following immune reconstitution from HAART
- ➢ Development of escape mutants
  - o Associated with use of lamivudine
  - o Clinical acute hepatitis
  - o Seroconversion to anti-HBe and/or HBs Ag
- ➢ HBV does not cause progression of HIV disease

Q6. What is the most common infections cause of *diarrhea* in HIV/AIDS patients in the HAART era?

A6.
- o C. Difficile
- o "punishment marks if you said Giardia lamblia or Entamoeba histolytica

Q7. Infections by *enteric bacteria* such as Salmonella, Shigella and Campylobacter are common and virulent in HIV/AIDS. Give their characteristics in this setting.

A7.
- o High rates of bacteremia
- o High rates of antibiotic resistance
- o May need to be treated with IV ciprofloxacin

Q8. What is the commonest cause of *drug-induced diarrhea* in HIV/AIDS?

A8. The commonest cause of drug-induced diarrhea in HIV/AIDS is HAART therapy (protease inhibitors), the most common of which for diarrhea as an adverse effect is Nelfinavir.

Q9. An HIV/AIDS patient develops bloody diarrhea, fever and a *raised serum LDH* concentration. What is the most likely infections cause?

A9. Histoplasmosis, causing diffuse colitis with ulceration.

Q10. What are the infectious agents which are most commonly induced in the *immune reconstitution* syndrome following the introduction of HAART therapy?

A10.
- Myobacteria, e.g. MAC lymphadenitis
- CMV, e.g. CMV uveitis

Q11. What is the viral infection associated with condyloma acuminatum and *squamous cell carcinoid* of the anorectal area in HIV/AIDS?

A11. HPV (human papilloma virus)

Q12. What is the *screening* method to detect this infection, and what do they predict?

A12. Cytological specimens of the anal canal are used to screen for HPV (type 16 and 18), and have a high predictive valve for dysplasia.

Q13. What general group of causes of *upper GI blood* (UGIB) is most frequently involved in HIV/AIDS patients in the HAART era?

A13. Causes of UGIB not related to HIV/AIDS are the comment cause in the HAART-treated patient.

Q14. What is the commonest cause of *lower GI bleeding* in HIV/AIDS patients in the HAART era?

A14. CMV colitis

Q15. Name three infections which *do not cause colitis* and rectal bleeding in HIV/AIDS?

A15. Pathogens which do not cause mucosal ulceration (such as MAC, microsporidia and cryptosporidia) do not cause bleeding.

Q16. Drug-induced liver injury (DILI) is common in HIV/AIDS treatment HAART (ritonavir is the most common). A hepatocellular biochemical pattern is seen. Indirect hyperbilirubinemia is uncommon except for indinavir. In this context, what is the *lactic acidosis syndrome*?

A16. The lactic acidosis syndrome

- The nucleoside reverse transcriptase inhibitors (eg., zidovudine, dideoxy inosine [ddI] and stavudine) reduce mitochondrial DNA synthesis.
- The reduced mitochondrial DNA synthesis leads to damage in
  - Liver
    - Hepatomegaly
    - Fatty liver
    - Liver failure
  - Pancreas
    - Pancreatitis
  - Muscle
    - Myopathy
  - Nerve
    - Peripheral neuropathy

Q17. In the context of HIV/AIDS, which infectious agents cause Kaposi sarcoma and bacillary peliosis hepatitis?

A17.
- Kaposi sarcoma – HHV-8 (human herpes virus-8)
- Bacillary peliosis hepatitis-Bartonella henselae, or quintana

## 2. Solid organ transplant

Q1. Give 4 unusual features of the postoperative course of kidney transplant, or *kidney/pancreas transplant.*

A1.
- GERD-develops in ~ 50%
  - Associated with ↑ kidney graft loss and death
- ↑ risk of HBV or HCV (~50%)
- Interferon α and ribavirin cannaot be used to treat HCV in KT (↑ risk of allograft rejection)
- ↑ risk of GI bleeding, with ↑ mortality rate
- ↑ risk of intestinal ischemia (especially KT for polycystic kidney disease)

Q2. About half of all persons having a transplantation of the heart (HT), lung (LT), or heart plus lung (HLT) will develop GI symptoms. Give 7 gi conditions which develop after *HT, LT or HLT.*

A2.
- Esophagus
  - GERD
  - Severe necrotizing fungal esophagitis, complicated with esophageal perforation
  - Increase the risk of obliterative bronchiolitis
- Stomach
  - Gastroparesis (possibly due to CMV V2V)
  - Giant (>3 cm) gastric ulcers (no ↑ risk of H. pylori infection)

| | |
|---|---|
| ➢ Bowel | ○ Diverticulitis<br>○ Ischemic colitis<br>○ Infectious colitis<br>- CMV<br>- C. difficile |
| ➢ Pancreas | ○ Pancreatitis |
| ➢ Galbladder | ○ Cholelithiasis |
| ➢ GVHD (graft-versus-host disease) | ○ Fever, skin rash, GI symptoms<br>○ Non infectious diarrhea may increase the incidence and the fatal outcome |

Q3. In the context of hematopoietic cell tranplantation (HCT), what is the *Typhlitis Syndrome*?

A3.
- Typhlitis
  - Characterized by cecal inflammation, friability, ulceration and edema in persons who are neutropenic
  - Usually caused by C. septicum
  - Often results in polymicrobial sepsin

Q4. Give 3 methods to diagnose *hepatic fungal infection* in HCT.

A4.
- Diagnostic imaging
  - Ct, MRI
- Serum fungal biomarker assays
  - Galactomannan
  - Glucan
- Liver biopsy
  - PCR
  - Culture

## 3. Gastrointestinal manifestations of systemic disease

Q1. About 15% of patients with *rheumatoid arthritis* (RA) have positive biochemical markers for liver disease.

Give 6 histological changes in the liver seen in RA.

A1.

- Fatty liver
- Kupffer cell hyperplasia
- Portal tract infiltration of mononuclear cells
- Hepatic necrosis
- Periportal fibrosis
- ↑ incidence (associated) AIH, PBC
- HCV patients
  - 75% become rheumatoid –factor positive, some of whom develop mixed cryoglobulinemia
  - These persons raarely have antibodies to CCP (anticyclic citralinated peptide, so do not have true RA)
- RA plus HBV, treated with anti-TNF therapy → severe flares of HBV
- Fatty syndrome (splenomegaly and neutropenia)
  - ↑ incidence of hepatomegaly and abnormal Les
- DILI
  - Anti-TNF therapy associated hepatic toxicity

## 4. Systemic lupus erythematosus (SLE)

Q1. Give 10 GI complications of SLE

A1.

- Mouth
  - Oral ulcer
- Esophagus
  - ↓ motility
  - GERD
- Stomach
  - Hypertrophic gastropathy
  - Gastritis
- Small bowel
  - Protein-losing enteropathy
  - Steatorrhea
  - PCI (pneumatosis cystoides inntestinalis)
- Colon
  - NEC (necrotizing enterocolitis)
  - Vasculitis – small vessels
- Pancreas
  - Pancreatitis
- Liver
  - Lobular hepatitis
  - Antinuclear antibodies (but not AIH [autoimmune hepatitis])
  - NRH (nodular regenerative hyperplasia)
  - Budd-Chiari syndrome
    - Lupus anticoagulants
    - Anticordiolipin antibodies
  - Fatty liver

Q2. Vasculitis leading to ischemic changes in the GI tract are common in SLE. Visceral angiography is not usually helpful in this setting. CT diagnostic imaging may help to make this diagnosis of ischemia in SLE.

Give the typical features of CT which help to make the diagnosis of bowel ischemia in SLE.

A2.

- Bowel wall thickened ± target sign
- Target sign (bowel wall thickening plus
  - Peripheral rim enhancement (hyperattenuation)
  - Inner and outer rim enhanced, with the centre not enhanced (hypoattenuation)
- Intestinal segments – dilation
- Mesenteric vessels – engaged
- Mesenteric fat – hyperattenuation

Q3.

- In SLE, the vasculitis is usually in the small vessels, and visceral angiography is not very useful diagnostically.
- In contrast, the vasculitis which occurs in polyarteritis nodosa (PAN) is a necrotizing vasculitis which involves both the small as well as the medium-sized arteries.
- In fact, about 80% of PAN patients will have aneurysmal dilations especially if the superior mesenteric artery.
- Thus, bowel ischemia is common.

Give 4 GI associations of *PAN* in addition to bowel ischemia, with its complications of infarction and perforation.

| | | |
|---|---|---|
| A3. | ➢ Gall bladder / BT | ○ Acalculous cholecystitis<br>○ Hemobilia<br>○ Biliary strictures |
| | ➢ Pancreas | ○ Pancreatis |
| | ➢ Liver | ○ Hepatic infarcts<br>○ HBV infection |

## 5. Polymyositis and dermatomyositis

Q1. Polymyositis and dermatomyositis have been traditionally considered to represent an inflammatory myopathy of skeletal muscle. This would explain transfer dysphagia and nasal regurgitation, but how is it explained that these patients may have other GI complications such as disorders of the motility of the lower esophagus, gastroporesis, and hypomotility of the small ntestine, pneumoitosis intestinalis, as well as colonic dilation and pseudodiverticula.

What is the explanation of the GI symptoms which develops in these parts of the GI tract which do not contain skeletal muscle.

A1. Involvement in polymyositis and dermatomyositis extents to GI tract smooth muscle, as well as the skeletal muscle in the upper third of the esophagus.

Q2. Polymyositis, PSS and SLE may overlap in a syndrome known as *MCTD* (mixed connective tissue damage).

What is the unusual therapeutic feature of the esophageal motility complication which occur in MCTD?

A2. In MCTD, the esophageal motility disorder responds to glucocorticosteroids.

Q3. *Churg-Strauss Syndrome* (CSS, aka allergic granulomatous angitis) is characterized by sinusitis, rhititis, asthma and peripheral eosinophilia.
Give 5 complications of CSS.

A3.

- Abdominal pain (nausea, vomiting, bleeding)
  - Eosinophilic gastroenteritis (diarrhea)
  - Ulcerations
  - Perforations
- Pancreas
  - Pancreatis
- Gallbladder
  - Cholecystitis
- Colon
  - Ulceration
- Peritoneum
  - Ascites

Q4. Henoch-Schonlein Purpura (HSP) is characterized by abdominal pain, renal disease, arthralgias and non-thrombocytopenic purpura arising from a systemic vasculitis. GI bleeding is also common. Give 6 GI complications of HSP, other than the abdominal pain and GI bleeding.

A4.

- Small bowel
  - Aphthous ulcers
  - Walll thickening
  - Dilation
  - Protein-losing enteropathy
  - Strictures
  - Intramural hematoma
  - Intussusceptions

- Colon — Ischemic perforations
- Appendix — Appendicitis
- Pancreas — Pancreatits
- Gallbladder — Cholecystitis

Q5. *Wegener's granulomatosis* (WG) is characterized by vasculitis involving sinuses, lung and kidney. When WG involves the GI tract, why may it be confused with Crohn disease (CD)?

A5. The GI complications of WG include

| | |
|---|---|
| Stomach | Granulomatous |
| Small bowel | Ileocolitis, with granulomas* - may mimic CD |
| Gallbladder | Gangrenous cholecystitis |
| Cryoglobulinemia | Mesenteric vasculitis (rare) |

Q6. Mixed cryoglobulinemia (raised serum concentration of IgG plus IgM) is characterized by arthralgia, purpura, and asthenia.

Give 5 GI *associations of cryoglobulinemia*

A6.

- HCV infection
- IBD
- Celiac disease
- Postintestinal bypass syndrome
- Small intestinal
  - Colonic vasculitis
  - Ischemia
  - Diarrhea
  - Perforation

Q7. *Behcet disease* (BD) is characterized by uvetis, aphthous ulcers of the mouth, skin lesions, and genital ulcers. About half of BD patients have GI complications which may mimic Crohn disease (CD).

Give GI complications of BD which reflect why BD needs to be differentiated from CD.

A7.

- Esophagus
    - Aphthous ulcer
    - Perforation
    - Varices
- Stomach
    - Aphthous ulcers
- Small bowel
    - Ulcers (punch-out)
    - Fistulas enteroenteric
- Colon
    - Punched-out ulcers
    - Fistulas
        - Perianal
        - Rectovaginal
- Liver
    - Budd-Chiari Syndrome (thrombosis of hepatic vein)
    - Portal vein thrombosis

Q8. A middle-aged man who moved to Canada 20 years ago from Lebanon develop acute abdominal pain, fever, arthralgias. The relapsing and remitting nature of the symptoms led to the consideration of porphyria as the diagnosis, but laboratory investigations for porphyria were negative. CT scan of the abdomen suggested small bowel obstruction. Give the *renal conditions* which may develop.

A8.

- Nephrotic syndrome
- Amyloidosis
- Chronic renal failure

Q9. I still do not know the diagnosis!

A9.
- The diagnosis is *familial mediterranean fever* (FMF), an autosomal recessive disease due to a disorder in the gene MEFV, leading to an abnormal protein, pyrin (aka marenostrin).
- With many of his attacks he would have developed sterile peritonitis, leading to the symptoms of small bowel obstruct from adhesions.
- Treatment is with colchicine.

## 6. Diabetes of gut

Q1. Give the role of EMG studies in the diabetic patient with unexplained *upper abdominal pain*.

A1. An abnormal EMG of the anterior abdominal wall muscles, as compared with an EMG of Thoracic paraspinal muscles, supports the diagnosis of diabetic radiculopathy (neuropathy of thoracic nerve roots)

## 7. Neuromuscular diseases affecting GI tract

Q1. GI symptoms are common (70%) in persons with multiple sclerosis (MS), such as oropharyngeal dysphagia.
Give 4 causes of constipation related to MS.

A1. Causes of constipation in patients with MS that are related to the MS include

- ↓ activity
- Rectal intussusception
- Rectal outlet obstruction
- Stercoral ulcers
- Incoordinated relaxation of muscles
  - Puborectalis
  - IAS (internal anal sphincter)

Q2. GI complications are common often a cardiovascular accident (CVA), or *injury to the head* or *spinal column*. Give 3 of the most common lesions.

A2. The numbers in brackets indicate the percentage of patients with these lesions seen on EGD.

- CVA, Head Injury
  - Esophagus
    - Esophagitis (11%)
  - Stomach
    - Gastritis (69%)
    - Gastric ulcer (23%)
  - Duodenum
    - Duodentis (8%)

Source: Feldman, M., et al. *Saunders/Elsevier* 2010, page 579.

- Spinal cord
  - Esophagus
    - GERD
  - Stomach
    - Gastroparasis
      - ↓ availability of drugs for absorption
    - Ulceration (GU)
  - Duodenum
    - Ulceration (DU)
      - ↑ risk of
        - Bleeding
        - Asymptomatic perforation
  - Small intestine
    - Amyloidosis (secondary)
  - Pancreas
    - Pancreatitis
  - Colon
    - Constipation
      - Sensation ↓ rectaal fullness
      - Motor ↓ control of defecation

Q3. Why is the *defecation reflex* usually intact in a person with spinal cord injury?

A3. The defecation reflex is usually intact in spinal cord injury patients because the lower motor neurons of the $S_2$, $S_3$ and $S_4$ sacral nerve roots.

Q4. Idiopathic *autonomic neuropathy* affecting the sympathetic and/or parasympathetic systems often (70%) affects the GI tract.

Give the symptoms which suggest autonomic (parasympathetic) neuropathy.

A4.

- Diarrhea
  - Hypersalvation
  - Hyperhydrosis
- *Note
  - Small intestinal bacterial overgrowth is uncommon, despite the common manometric demonstration of motility disorders associated with some neurological disorders such as CVA

## 8. Amyloidosis

Q1. The liver commonly involved in primary amyloidosis, and the GI tract in secondary amyloidosis (classification systems now stress the different types of fibrillar proteins in the amyloid deposits, rather than the primary and secondary designations). The GI tract can be affected from the mouth to the anus, as well as the liver, pancreas and spleen. Depending upon where the amyloid is deposited in the GI tract will determine the nature of the symptoms:

Give the *clinical presentations* when mayloid affects different parts of the wall of the intestine.

A1.
- Muscularis mucosa
  - ↓ absorption
- Muscle layer
  - Dysmotility
- Vessel walls
  - Ischemia
  - Infarction
- Direct pressure damage to myenteric plexus and visceral nerve trunks

**9. ICU – Type patient**

Q1. Hepatic dysfunction is common in patients with *systemic infections* arising from diverticulitis, appendicitis, lobar pneumonia, or pyelonephritis. The biochemical profile usually reflects underlying cholestasis which is associated with sepsis or extrahepatic infection.

Give the changes seen on liver biopsy of a patient with systemic infection.

A1. The changes on liver biopsy of a patient with systemic infection include:

- Hepatocytes
  - Little changes, no necrosis
  - Portal area
    - Mild portal infiltrate of mononuclear cells
  - Some parenchymal dropot
- Zone 2 and 3
  - Bile stasis
- Cholanitis lenta
  - Dlated
  - Bile thrombi
  - Surrounded by neutrophils
- Mild steatosis
- Mild Kupffer cell hyperplasia

**References and Suggested Reading**


1. Baliga RR. 250 Cases in Clinical Medicine. *Saunders/Elsevier*, Philadelphia 2007.
2. Burton JL. Aids to Postgraduate Medicine. *Churchill Livingstone*, Edinburgh, 1971.
3. Davey P. Medicine at a Glance. 2nd edition, *Wiley-Blackwell*, Malden, Mass, 2006.
4. Davies IJT. Postgraduate Medicine *Lloyd-Luke (medical books) LTD* 1972.
5. El-serag HB. ACG Annual Postgraduate Course: 2009
6. Filate W, Leung R, Ng D, and Sinyor M. Essentials of Clinical Examination Handbook. 5th Edition. *The Medical Society, Faculty of Medicine, University of Toronto*, 2005.
7. Fledman, M., et al. Sleisenger and Fordtran's Gastrointestinal and Liver Disease. 9th Edition. *Saunders/Elsevier*, Philadephia, 2010.
8. Grey J, Ed. Therapeutic Choices. 6th Edition, *Canadian Pharmacists Association, Ottawa,* 2012.
9. Jugovic PJ, Bitar R, and McAdam LC. Fundamental Clinical Situations: A Practical OSCE Study Guide. 4th Edition. *Saunders/ Elsevier*, Toronto, Canada, 2004.
10. Mangione S. Physical Diagnosis Secrets. *Hanley & Belfus*, Philadelphia, 2000.
11. McGee SR. Evidence Based Physical Diagnosis. 2nd Edition. *Saunders/Elsevier*, St.Louis, Missouri, 2007.
12. Simel DL, Rennie Drummond, Keitz Sheri A. The Rational Clinical Examination: Evidence- based clinical diagnosis. *JAMA* 2009.
13. Spiegel, BMR, et al. Acing the Hepatology Questions on the GI Board Exam: The Ultimate Crunch-Time Resource. *Slack Incorporated* 2011.
14. Talley NJ, et al. Clinical Examination: a Systematic Guide to Physical Diagnosis. *Maclennan & Petty Pty Limited*, East gardens, Australia, 2003

**Useful Websites**

1. http://gi.org/
2. http://www.aasld.org/Pages/Default.aspx
3. http://www.bsg.org.uk/
4. http://www.cag-acg.org/
5. http://www.easl.eu/
6. http://www.gastro.org/
7. http://www.worldgastroenterology.org/
8. www.expertconsult.com
9. www.hepatology.ca

## Index

www.ingramcontent.com/pod-product-compliance
Lightning Source LLC
Chambersburg PA
CBHW051441170526
45166CB00001B/71

* 9 7 8 1 4 7 8 2 9 5 3 6 5 *